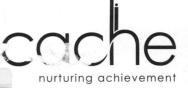

nurturing achievement

# The EYFS

## A Practical Guide for Students and Professionals

Vicky Hutchin

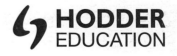

**HODDER**
EDUCATION

Orders: please contact Bookpoint Ltd, 130 Milton Park, Abingdon, Oxon OX14 4SB. Telephone: (44) 01235 827720. Fax: (44) 01235 400454. Lines are open from 9.00–5.00, Monday to Saturday, with a 24-hour message answering service. You can also order through our website **www.hoddereducation.co.uk**

*British Library Cataloguing in Publication Data*
A catalogue record for this title is available from the British Library

ISBN: 978 1 4441 5741 3

This Edition Published 2012
Impression number    10 9 8 7 6 5 4 3 2
Year                              2015, 2014, 2013, 2012

Hachette UK's policy is to use papers that are natural, renewable and recyclable products and made from wood grown in sustainable forests. The logging and manufacturing processes are expected to conform to the environmental regulations of the country of origin.

Cover photo © Alena Ozerova – Fotolia

Typeset by Pantek Media, Maidstone Kent
Printed and bound in Italy for Hodder Education, An Hachette UK Company, 338 Euston Road, London NW1 3BH.

# Contents

# Acknowledgements

I would like to give a very special thanks to all the settings and schools, practitioners, children and parents, who have contributed so much to this book. A special mention goes to the settings and schools who so generously gave me their time as the book developed, and the discussions which turned into the case studies:

Peter Catling and the staff team at Woodlands Park Nursery School and Children's Centre, London;

Joyce Clark and the staff team at St Anne's Nursery School & Children's Centre, London;

Ludmila Morris and the staff team at McMillan Nursery School and Children's Centre Hillingdon;

Pat Davies, Karen Wishart, Jess Snell, Donna Harvey and the staff team at Chingford Hall Primary School and Children's Centre, Waltham Forest;

Veronica Larocque, Pat Lee and Kelly Hayes at Fiveways Playcentre, Brighton;

Wendy Plater and the staff team at Bright Start Nursery, Brighton;

Marcelo Staricoff, Robb Johnson and Michelle Connolly and the staff team at Hertford Infants School, Brighton;

Thanks are also due to Michelle Barrett and staff at Vanessa Nursery School, London.

And a very special thanks to Kerry, Dave, Mary, Becky, Josh, Maria Paula, Esteban, Fran, James, Mary and Jonathan.

As always, a very special thank you to Billy Ridgers, who took many of the photographs and read and commented on copious drafts. This book would not have happened without his unconditional support and time. I would also like to thank Colin Goodlad and Chloé Harmsworth at Hodder Education for their support in getting this project off the ground, and to Andrew Callaghan for his photographs.

All photos © Andrew Callaghan, except:

Figures: 1.5, 1.7, 2.4, 3.8, 3.13, 3.14, 3.15, 3.16, 3.17, 3.18, 3.19, 4.3, 5.1, 5.2, 5.7, 7.9, 8.1, 8.6, 8.7, 10.1, 10.3a & b, 10.4, 11.7, 11.8, 12.1, 13.2a & b, 14.1, 14.3, 15.5, 15.6 © Billy Ridgers.

# Introduction

*"A child is not a vase to be filled but a candle to be lit"* François Rabelais

This book focuses on learning and development in the early years. The framework for early years in England, the Early Years Foundation Stage (EYFS), first became statutory in 2008 and was revised in 2012. The quotation above, written in the early 16th Century, was quoted in the initial review report on the Early Years Foundation Stage (EYFS) in 2011 by Dame Clare Tickell. (Tickell, 2011). It expresses the beliefs that underpin the EYFS and provides us with a great way to think about our work with young children.

The learning and development that takes place in the first five years of life is greater and more rapid than at any other time in life. Those of us in the lucky position of working with young children or being students of childcare and education are privileged to have such a great job, contributing to children's learning and development. It is so exciting when we are tuned in and our minds are open, receptive to what we see and hear.

James started at nursery when he was aged 3 years 4 months. From his first week he loved to be outside playing firefighters with a small group of other children. Before he started his mother had told his key person how fond he was of a cartoon about a firefighter, so the nursery knew to put out the firefighter helmets and set up a pretend fire station. His play was very active, moving fast around the garden and up and down the climbing frame with fire helmet on, using the resources and equipment supplied for the play by the practitioners.

10 months later, he continued to be interested in similar play themes based on cartoons he loved to watch on DVD or television. He was now able make his own props for his play: paper capes, maps, swords and shields out of cardboard. In the process he developed a range of skills for using tools such as scissors, hole punchers, tape dispensers and pens to help him. His play had a more complex storyline now and he was able to tell others who wanted to be involved what roles they could play.

In the 10 months between the two observations, he was helped in his learning and development by the practitioners in the nursery, in close partnership with his family. The effective support he was given in the nursery was based on the practitioners' knowledge of child development and learning, their knowledge about him as an individual and their skills in applying their knowledge. They used what he was passionate about to help him use his rich imagination, developing his ideas and skills at expressing them. This provided him with the motivation to try out new skills, such as drawing, cutting and joining. His tentative mark making from 10 months earlier had developed into confident representations of people and writing-like marks, including the first letter of his name.

## The Early Years Foundation Stage

This book is designed to help professionals and students working in the early years to support children to the best of their abilities, just as happened with James. The good thing is that the EYFS provides the backing for this approach. Since it was first introduced in 2008 it took its lead from the very best practice in England, backed up by evidence from well respected UK and international research on children's learning and development. The revised version in 2012 has continued in this vein, building on what was already available.

The EYFS encompasses all aspects of practice and is for *everyone* who works with children outside the child's home environment. When the EYFS was first published in 2007 there was much acclaim for the themes and principles which so clearly set out what we need to consider in providing the best for children. The EYFS review report in 2011 by Dame Clare Tickell (Tickell 2011) acknowledged how useful these have been. They continue to be as important as ever and are often referred to by primary and even secondary school headteachers and senior managers as something they also believe is right for the pupils and students in their schools.

## Diversity and inclusion

Throughout the book there are case studies demonstrating highly effective EYFS practice in a range of different early childhood settings. These are here to support the reader in thinking about what they might do in their own settings. Some particularly focus on inclusion and all the settings in the case studies place inclusion at the heart of their practice. There are copious observations of children learning and developing across the age range in every chapter, taken by practitioners and parents. These observations help the reader understand what children's learning and development looks like, demonstrating the uniqueness and amazing abilities of *every* child and their individual journeys in learning and development.

## The structure of the book

Each chapter is structured in the same way, to guide the reader logically and easily through each topic:

- **What the EYFS tells us.** Each chapter begins with a section explaining the EYFS theme or topic to be considered.
- **Looking at children.** In this section of each chapter you will find observations of two different children. Over the course of the book, the full EYFS age range is covered, from young babies to five year olds. The observations demonstrate the uniqueness and diversity of children's interests, development and learning, related to the topic of the chapter. Each observation is analysed, to draw out what the observation shows us about the child's learning and development. Other examples of children learning are also threaded through the chapters.
- **What the experts say.** The work of one or two 'experts' in the field is discussed to support understanding of how children learn and show how theory and research helps us improve quality in practice.
- **Effective practice: what do we need to do?** This section highlights what we need to do to ensure the very best for the children. Most chapters end with a case study showing how practitioners in a particular setting are implementing effective, inclusive and *reflective* practice.

- **Activities:** Each chapter includes four activities. These provide opportunities to learn more about how children learn, help the reader to reflect on and review the EYFS practice in their setting, or provide ideas for activities to carry out with children.

The book is in five sections, each section is dedicated to a particular aspect of the EYFS.

| The Early Years Foundation Stage: Themes and Commitments | | | |
|---|---|---|---|
| **A Unique Child** | **Positive Relationships** | **Enabling Environments** | **Learning and Development** |
| **1.1 Child Development** Babies and children develop in individual ways and at varying rates. Every area of development – physical, cognitive, linguistic, spiritual, social and emotional – is equally important. | **2.1 Respecting Each Other** Every interaction is based on caring professional relationships and respectful acknowledgement of the feelings of children and their families. | **3.1 Observation, Assessment and Planning** Babies and young children are individuals first, each with a unique profile of abilities. Schedules and routines should flow with the child's needs. All planning starts with observing children in order to understand and consider their current interests, development and learning. | **4.1 Play and Exploration** Children's play reflects their wide ranging and varied interests and preoccupations. In their play children learn at their highest level. Play with peers is important for children's development. |
| **1.2 Inclusive Practice** The diversity of individuals and communities is valued and respected. No child or family is discriminated against. | **2.2 Parents as Partners** Parents are children's first and most enduring educators. When parents and practitioners work together in early years settings, the results have a positive impact on children's development and learning. | **3.2 Supporting Every Child** The environment supports every child's learning through planned experiences and activities that are challenging but achievable. | **4.2 Active Learning** Children learn best through physical and mental challenges. Active learning involves other people, objects, ideas and events that engage and involve children for sustained periods. |
| **1.3 Keeping Safe** Young children are vulnerable. They develop resilience when their physical and psychological well-being is protected by adults. | **2.3 Supporting Learning** Warm, trusting relationships with knowledgeable adults support children's learning more effectively than any amount of resources. | **3.3 The Learning Environment** A rich and varied environment supports children's learning and development. It gives them the confidence to explore and learn in secure and safe, yet challenging, indoor and outdoor spaces. | **4.3 Creativity and Critical Thinking** When children have opportunities to play with ideas in different situations and with a variety of resources, they discover connections and come to new and better understandings and ways of doing things. Adult support in this process enhances their ability to think critically and ask questions. |
| **1.4 Health and Well-being** Children's health is an integral part of their emotional, mental, social, environmental and spiritual well-being and is supported by attention to these aspects. | **2.4 Key Person** A key person has special responsibilities for working with a small number of children, giving them the reassurance to feel safe and cared for and building relationships with their parents. | **3.4 The Wider Context** Working in partnership with other settings, other professionals and with individuals and groups in the community supports children's development and progress towards the outcomes of *Every Child Matters*: being healthy, staying safe, enjoying and achieving, making a positive contribution and economic well-being. | **4.4 Areas of Learning and Development** The Early Years Foundation Stage (EYFS) is made up of seven areas of Learning and Development. All areas of Learning and Development are connected to one another and are equally important. All areas of Learning and Development are underpinned by the Principles of the EYFS. |
| department for education and skills | ISBN 978-1-84478-886-6 | | |

EYFS themes and commitments (DCSF 2008)

## Section 1: Understand the EYFS themes and principles

The themes and principles of the EYFS form a great starting point for the book. They underpin the work of early childhood professionals and influence not only the types of experiences and activities we offer to the children but *how* we offer them too.

The 2012 Statutory Framework for the EYFS reaffirms these overarching principles, although slightly changing the wording. The non-statutory Development Matters guidance uses the themes as the underpinning structure to the statements about what learning may look like, what adults can do, and what they can provide to support children's learning and development.

The first four chapters of the book consider one theme and principle and an explanation of the 'commitments', which were originally produced as a core part of the EYFS 2008 guidance. These describe effective practice and underpin the principles. They remain as important as ever (see page vii). In Chapter 4, Learning and Development we begin to look at *how* as well as *what* children are learning and why some areas of learning are called 'prime areas of learning' and others 'specific areas of learning'. Chapter 5 is devoted to a key aspect of the early years practitioner's work: *Developing strong partnership with parents and carers*. This is an area which was highlighted in the Tickell Review of the EYFS in 2011 as an area for development nationally.

## Section ll: The Characteristics of Learning – how children learn

The EYFS highlights three '**characteristics of effective learning**' which describe *how* children learn. They are the lifelong characteristics which help us to be successful learners, formed from the first three commitments of the theme Learning and Development. Each chapter in this section of the book takes a characteristic, explains what it is about and how practitioners can effectively facilitate and extend children's learning and development. Assessing the characteristics of learning is part of the statutory assessment of children alongside the 7 areas of learning, at the end of the reception year in school. This provides important information to pass on to the child's Year 1 teacher to help them plan appropriately for the children. It is also important that the characteristics are considered in assessment throughout the EYFS age range.

## Section lll: The Prime Areas of Learning

The three prime areas of learning form the topics for the chapters in Section lll. As the Tickell Review Report in 2011 stated:

*"It is widely agreed by researchers and practitioners that personal social and emotional development, physical development and communication and language are closely linked to one another and central to all other areas of learning and development"*

(Tickell, 2011).

## Section lV: The Specific Areas of Learning

Next we turn to the four specific areas of learning. The specific areas relate to the things we *want* children to learn, rather than to child development and each has a chapter of its own.

## Section V: Assessment in the EYFS

The final section of the book comprises just one very important chapter: **Assessing Children's Learning**. The chapter takes a deeper look both at the importance of observation and assessment in planning to meet the needs of the children (formative assessment) and how to summarise assessment from time to time. It includes information about how to prepare for the **progress check at age 2** to be shared with parents.

### Terminology

Throughout this book, the term 'parents' will be used to refer to children's main carers, usually, but not always, the biological parents. As EYFS 2008 stated: "Families are all different. Children may live with one or both parents, with other relatives or carers, with same-sex parents or in an extended family". The extended family may include grandparents, aunts, uncles, and for some children there may be other combinations too – for example, a parent living with a partner who is not the parent and the partner's children.

## Further reading and references

*Development Matters in the Early Years Foundation Stage* (2012). Available for download from: www.early-education.org.uk

The Foundation Years website has a range of materials for parents and practitioners including EYFS associated guidance documents: www.foundationyears.org.uk

*The Statutory Framework for the Early Years Foundation Stage: Setting the standards for learning, development and care for children from birth to five.* Available for download from: www.education.gov.uk

Tickell, C. (2011) *The Early Years: Foundations for Life, Health and Learning. An Independent Report on the Early Years Foundation Stage to Her Majesty's Government.* Available for download from: www.education.gov.uk

# Section 1: Understanding the EYFS themes and principles

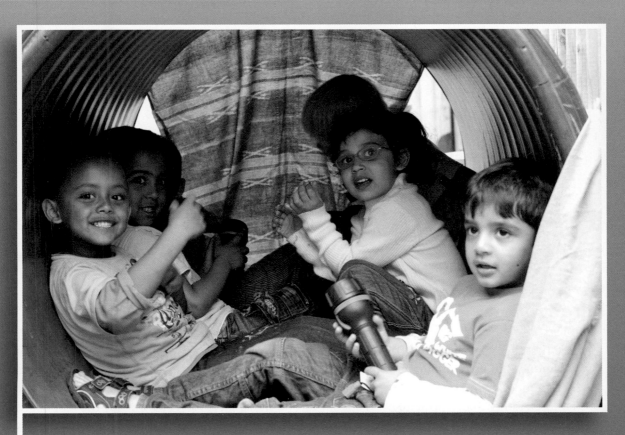

The themes, principles and commitments form the heart of the Early Years Foundation Stage (EYFS), emphasising that effective practice is based on sound principles that enable all professionals involved with children to provide the best quality experiences for them.

The themes are:
➤ A Unique Child (Chapter 1)
➤ Positive Relationships (Chapter 2)
➤ Enabling Environments (Chapter 3)
➤ Learning and Development (Chapter 4).

Each theme has a set of four supporting commitments, which set out in more detail important aspects of the principle.

The first four chapters in Section 1 explain the four principles and the commitments related to the themes. The final chapter in this section, Chapter 5 Developing strong partnerships with parents and carers, looks at one of these commitments in greater depth.

The EYFS principles and commitments are shown on page vii.

# Chapter 1

# A Unique Child

## In this chapter we will be looking at:

➤ the commitments for A Unique Child, paying particular attention to Child development and Inclusive practice

➤ observations of children as they learn and develop in their own ways, supported by their families and practitioners

➤ what some key experts say in relation to two of the commitments: Inclusive practice and Health and well-being

➤ what we do to ensure our practice is effective, with a case study on how one setting makes their provision stimulating, challenging and safe for children.

## Introduction

The first theme of the EYFS is 'A Unique Child'. As you will see in this chapter, the principle of A Unique Child sets the tone for the EYFS with a truly positive perspective about children and childhood. This permeates every element of the EYFS. But let us start by thinking about some children rather than a principle: it is late spring and the small garden area outside the hall-based pack-away playgroup is full of snails. Snails, because of their very nature and the fact that they move slowly, provide a wonderful opportunity for children to investigate. Some snails have been placed into a clear plastic container for the children to look more closely. The children are between the ages of 2 years 6 months and just over 3 years old.

*Several children became absorbed in watching, touching or picking up the snails. Each child took a different approach to the experience. Laura was keen to handle the snails. Ben was fascinated by the snails crawling on top of each other: "They're all cuddling", he said. Jack was fascinated by the difference in size and the number of snails in the container. Afterwards he decided to draw what he had seen: "I've drawn big and little snails…12 snails."*

(Hutchin, 2003)

Although they appear to be exploring together, each child is interested in a different aspect of the snails and snail behaviour. Their learning from this experience is personal and unique to each of them.

## The EYFS principle, A Unique Child, tells us:

*"Every child is a unique child, who is constantly learning and can be resilient, capable, confident and self-assured."*

(EYFS, 2012)

One of the most delightful elements of working with young children and babies is their individuality – no two children are the same; they think differently and respond to what they experience in different ways, just as adults do. We may have a lot in common with others around us, and for much of our time we want to be with others, but each of us is unique. Children are born into a particular context, which is hugely significant to them: the family context comes first and with it the culture of home, what is valued, appreciated and celebrated, as well as what is prohibited, frowned upon or ignored. Next comes the wider context and environment – not just the physical environment, but the people in the community that the family interacts with, including you and the other practitioners in your setting.

These individual experiences help to create a child's uniqueness.

*"Each child's personal story is important and is the starting point for supporting their learning and development."*

(EYFS, 2008)

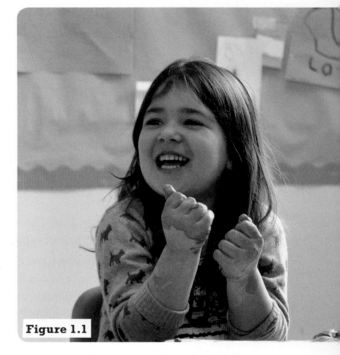

**Figure 1.1**

To provide the right support for every child we need to see them as unique, ensuring we address their individual needs and celebrate their individuality – what an exciting challenge this is! Child development may show us the most likely patterns of development that we expect to see for the majority of children, but – and this is important – it does not tell us the individual path each child will take.

## What is this theme about?

When we believe that every child is a competent learner, we are starting in the right place, as this encourages us to have high expectations and to work out how to help this come to fruition. Children with profound disabilities are just as competent learners as other children. When we get to know the children really well we can do more than just help them to fulfil what we think is their potential; we can *build on* their potential.

The principle tells us that children can be resilient, capable, confident and self-assured. They *can* be – with our help. Research has shown that close, positive relationships with caring adults in the early years builds the positive dispositions children need for their future lives. Developing positive relationships with the child and their family helps us to achieve this. Looking back at

James, who we met in the Introduction, it was finding out about his interests from his parents that helped the practitioners in the nursery to respond to him as a unique individual and to provide the stimulating environment that helped him gain confidence and develop new skills.

The four supporting commitments within A Unique Child are:
- Child development
- Inclusive practice
- Keeping safe
- Health and well-being.

## Child development

*"Babies and children develop in individual ways and at varying rates. Every area of development – physical, cognitive, linguistic, spiritual, social and emotional – is equally important."*

(EYFS card 1.1)

Having a good understanding of child development and learning is essential if we are to support children effectively. We can all too easily cut across and hinder their learning if we do not know enough.

From the moment of birth young babies begin to make sense of the new world they have just joined. They do this not only through using all their senses, but through the very close relationships they build with others, especially their mothers. Development and learning, though closely linked and dependent on each other, are different. Child development describes the patterns, sequences and pathways that most children take as they mature. Learning describes *how* children (and adults) acquire particular skills, knowledge and understanding, and attitudes, as well as *what* they learn. There are wide variations between children in the timings at which key developments may take place – for example, in being able to walk. You may well know of babies who walked at 9 or 10 months and others who did not walk until 18 months or more. However, this tells us nothing about their subsequent physical development or prowess at running, jumping, doing cartwheels or playing physical games later on.

### Activity

#### Thinking about child development

Compare two children of similar ages in your setting. What are the similarities and differences between them? For example:
- their interests and passions
- what they choose to play with and how
- differences in how they communicate
- their physical skills
- how they respond to others.

## Links to the EYFS areas of learning

The commitment statement on child development lists five aspects of development (*physical, cognitive, linguistic, spiritual, social* and *emotional*) and these are generally accepted to cover all aspects of body and brain development. The EYFS areas of learning not only cover all aspects of child development, but also what we want children to be learning in the seven areas of the EYFS. In Sections 3 and 4 we look in detail at each of the areas of learning and development in turn.

## Inclusive practice

*"The diversity of individuals and communities is valued and respected. No child or family is discriminated against".*

(EYFS card 1.2)

Inclusive practice is at the heart of effective practice because being inclusive means we are doing the best for everyone. Striving to be truly inclusive is one of the great joys of working in the early years. It gives us a real positive buzz as we celebrate the diversity among us and develop a sense of community and belonging. Being inclusive also ensures we have high expectations of every child and is vital to the future life chances of the children.

The starting point is listening to parents talk about their children: how energising this is when we are able to get into good conversations with parents about what their children do at home, the people who are important to them, the languages they speak, as well as what they like and don't like. Knowing about the things children do at home and what parents feel broadens the way we think, opening our minds to the many different ways of doing things, as well as helping us to share and celebrate our similarities. But the opposite of inclusion is exclusion. In very many ways our society is not fair, so trying to make it fairer through the way we work with children and families is really important. Certain groups of people are at risk of being disadvantaged and excluded as a result of a whole host of factors over which they have no control. This includes ethnicity, culture, religion, home language, family background, gender, learning difficulties and disabilities.

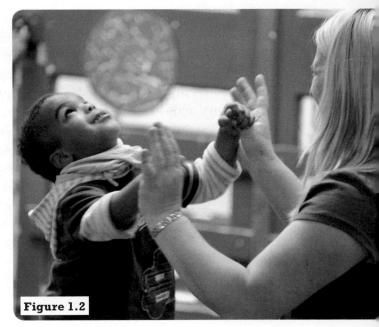

**Figure 1.2**

We know from national statistics collected on the Early Years Foundation Stage Profile (for example, from 2007–11) that year after year social and economic disadvantage, ethnicity, gender and learning English as an additional language all make a difference to outcomes for children. Boys do not do as well as girls, and certain minority ethnic groups, especially children who suffer most from poverty and racism, do not do nearly as well as white British children.

Children from the poorest backgrounds have much lower outcomes than others, and in 2010, for example, there was a difference of nearly 20 percentage points. Yet these children are no less intelligent or competent.

What we do day by day, moment by moment with the children in early years settings is vital to their success: they learn from everything around them, the negative as well as the positive, so you can see how vital it is to work against discrimination. Children soak up negative attitudes about themselves, their families and other people just as easily as the positive ones, so we need to create a positive, inclusive and fair environment. The UK is culturally and ethnically diverse, with families from all over the globe, giving us a great opportunity to take advantage of this and find out more about cultures, diversity and similarities between us, especially if this diversity is not reflected in your setting or part of the country. A fair environment is one in which everyone can achieve beyond their potential. It is a better environment for everyone – children, parents, practitioners, students and visitors alike.

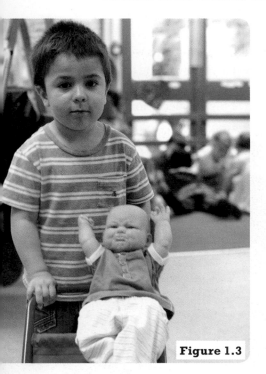

**Figure 1.3**

To achieve all this we have real backing through the EYFS. Not only is there the Inclusive Practice commitment, but there is also a legal requirement to act against discrimination, ensure equality of opportunity and have a written policy to promote it. There are also statutory duties, of course, and it is up to us to develop the very best practice for every child to have an exciting, enjoyable experience.

There is a great deal we can do to make sure our settings are inclusive and this starts by reflecting on your own setting's practice to find out how well you are doing. What do the parents think? What do children think? What about the wider community around your setting – would every child and family be equally welcomed and able to participate fully? If a new family arrived into your area, perhaps a refugee family who do not yet speak English, would they be welcomed too? These are all things we need to think about and reflect on when considering how inclusive our practice and provision really is.

## Activity

### How inclusive are your setting's resources and displays?

- How do the resources in your setting reflect diversity? Start by looking at the books on display. Do they reflect and celebrate diversity and inclusion? Do they show children from different ethnic origins as main characters as well as children with disabilities? Are there books about boys in caring roles and girls in active roles?
- Do you have a good supply of dressing-up clothes for boys, apart from firefighters, policemen, etc.?
- Does your home corner kitchen equipment reflect diversity?
- Are girls and boys encouraged to play in all areas of the setting?
- Check any posters, puzzles, games and displays that contain photographs or images of people: do they show diversity of gender, ethnicity, children with disabilities and special needs?

# Keeping safe

*"Young children are vulnerable. They develop resilience when their physical and psychological well-being is protected by adults."*

(EYFS card 1.3)

The keeping safe commitment reflects closely the requirements of the EYFS Statutory Framework Safeguarding and Welfare Requirements, particularly the sections on safeguarding, suitable people and staff ratios, taking medication, health, behaviour, safety and suitability of premises, environment and equipment, and outings. It is essential that when we work with the children we are fully aware of and adhere to these requirements since they are there for good reason. Young children are competent but do not yet have the knowledge, skills and understanding they need to keep themselves safe, which means they are vulnerable and need careful protection. We have made great strides in keeping children safe in recent years, but things can go wrong, and when they do the consequences can be devastating.

It is important to be aware of the difference between a danger or hazard and a risk. A danger or hazard can cause harm, but there may be a low or high risk that the hazard will cause harm. We need to be alert to possible hazards and dangers and take steps to eradicate the risks. For example, having a pond may seem a great enhancement educationally to an environment, but could be very hazardous to the children. A fence around the pond in the garden that children can see through reduces the risk of falling in. Taking only two or three children at a time into the enclosure under full adult supervision enables children to look closely or go pond dipping and to benefit from the experience safely. As Jennie Lindon tells us, "Everyone needs to remember the main goal: that children are enabled to move towards being competent and confident adults." (1999).

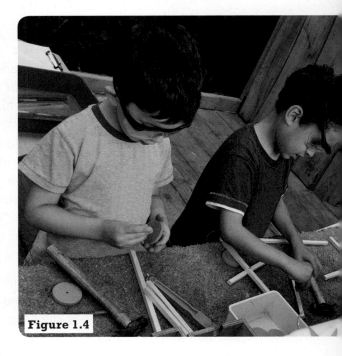

**Figure 1.4**

However, we must also make sure that we offer children plenty of exciting opportunities and challenges – being safe does not mean being unimaginative, boring or limiting. Children need to learn to take risks *safely*. If children are wrapped up in cotton wool and constantly told not to do certain things, we are storing up problems for them later in life. They will grow up not understanding how to be independent and unable to assess risks for themselves. Luckily, over the last few years there has been a realisation at national level that children were not able to be outside enough in safe but interesting outdoor environments. Recent developments have meant that many settings are now able to provide more challenging spaces, resources and equipment, which help children understand the power of their own muscles and understand risk.

In some of the photographs in this book you will see children of 3 years and upwards doing what seem like risky things. This has been possible because risk assessments have been made and the children have been taught the basic safety rules and are frequently reminded of them. The children doing woodwork have been shown how to hold the tools and equipment, where to stand and the importance of safety goggles to protect their eyes. Wonderful and challenging environments can be created for children, making it possible for them to climb trees, climb a challenging climbing wall and swing from monkey bars. However, before any of these things were made available to the children, a careful risk assessment was carried out and local authority safety regulations were adhered to.

## Health and well-being

*"Children's health is an integral part of emotional, mental, social and spiritual well-being and is supported by attention to these aspects."*

(EYFS card 1.4)

Healthy development is not just about ensuring that the environment is safe, clean and free from hazards, and that food is nutritious (for example, having fruit rather than biscuits for a snack); it is also about promoting the children's well-being. Well-being affects how we learn: if we are feeling uncomfortable, insecure or anxious, we cannot function properly or take on board new ideas and new experiences. Children learn when their well-being is high and this is at its height when they are relaxed, having fun and thoroughly enjoying what they are doing.

Having fun is an integral part of learning. It helps children to be creative, use their imagination and develop resilience and self-assurance: all things that the EYFS promotes. This means making sure that all the experiences and activities you provide are enjoyable and that you enter into the spirit of the children's explorations and interests with them.

For their health and well-being, children need plenty of opportunities for active play and encouragement to use their creativity and imagination. They need to be outside as much as possible, being physically active, getting plenty of fresh air – while suitably dressed for the weather, of course! This is not only important for their physical development, but it also impacts on brain development, thinking skills, learning and all aspects of well-being. If children are restrained because the environment or activities provided do not allow them to move as they need to, their learning and development will be adversely affected.

The close, warm and supportive relationships you form with the children are key to creating their emotional well-being too. Helping children to express their own feelings of discomfort and frustration, as well as joy and happiness, is all part of creating the kind of provision that is just right for every child.

# Looking at children:
## What do we see?

### Dreem, age 2 years 7 months

We see Dreem in these observations in his first week in the under-threes provision in a Children's Centre where he attends 15 hours a week. During the week his key person, Jenny, noticed his interest in the garden, in particular digging. He used a trowel and a small fork to dig out the weeds for the planter. At the sand tray he used the scoops and spades, pouring dry sand from one to the other. It was becoming clear to Jenny that his interest was not in the gardening so much as in the tools. She also noticed how keen he was to join in with cutting up the fruit for snack using a knife.

### What have we found out?

At first it appeared that Dreem's interest was in gardening, but by observing him in different situations over his first few days it was clear that his interest was in using real tools and participating in activities that adults usually do, such as cutting fruit or digging the garden. Jenny shares her plans for him with his mother. As he enjoys using tools to cut, dig and scoop she will provide more opportunities, such as putting out knives with the playdough and using scissors.

### Rosie, age 3 years 5 months

Rosie is 10 months older than Dreem and goes to a different setting. Like Dreem, she has only started attending the setting recently. In this observation, sand in individual sand trays has been put out on the table, with very small containers, tiny scoops and teaspoons. To begin with, Rosie seems more interested in the texture of the sand than using the equipment. She rubs her hands together, noticing bubbles appearing as she rubs (there is washing-up liquid in the sand). "Bubbles," she says. "It feels wet."

As she continues to explore the texture she begins to tell the practitioner about how she went trick or treating (it is just after Halloween) and how she dressed up as a witch. Then she starts to fill one of the small metal cups in the sand tray. "I made a birthday cake. I had some fairy cupcakes for my birthday – strawberry ones. I'm making cupcakes now. Mine's feeling bubblier." As she scoops the sand out she touches the bottom of the sand tray. "It's a bit warm," she says, noticing the difference between the temperature of the tray and the sand.

### What have we found out?

Both Rosie and Dreem's play involves using sand, but they play in very different ways unique to their individual interests. Rosie is interested in the texture of the sand, whereas Dreem is more interested in the tools and equipment. Rosie is able to describe confidently what she notices, and the language she uses shows her understanding of how language works (from "bubbles" to "bubblier"). She enjoys sharing information about her life with others.

As the staff plan what opportunities and possibilities to provide next for Rosie, they are well aware of her interest in materials and textures, and other observations note how she loves to play with cornflour, soapfoam and water, as well as sand.

## What the experts say
### Inclusive practice and well-being

### Developing inclusive practice

Babette Brown has worked tirelessly to help practitioners and students to find the best ways to combat discrimination and to work in an inclusive way. She has written a number of helpful books and made several DVDs, with plenty of ideas for practitioners to help children understand fairness and be inclusive. She stresses the importance of "giving children the opportunities to learn about and value each other's cultures, languages and abilities and lifestyles as this enables them to draw strength from their own". As she says in the introduction to her first book *Unlearning Discrimination in the Early Years* (1999): "As educators we know that young children are profoundly influenced by their families and by the communities in which they live but we may be less aware of the part that social factors like racism, sexism, social class, homophobia and ableism play in their lives." The book provides a wealth of practical ways to develop the way you work with children. For example, in a section entitled "An opportunity to rate yourself", Babette Brown provides a useful checklist of questions to help practitioners gauge how inclusive their provision really is.

In 2001 Brown set up the charity, Persona Doll Training UK. The Persona Doll approach helps practitioners to find meaningful ways to talk with young children about inclusion, fairness and unfairness, and through this to support their developing confidence and self-esteem. The practitioner uses a doll to tell stories about the doll's life; in addition to stories portraying the doll's positive life experiences, the unfair and discriminatory events in the child's life are presented. The children are asked to come up with solutions to the problem for the doll. This approach is used around the world, including Europe, the USA, Southeast Asia, Australia and South Africa.

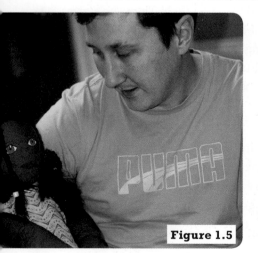

**Figure 1.5**

In her book *Equality in Action*, published in 2008, Babette evaluates research (including her own) on the impact of Persona Dolls in supporting the development of inclusive practice.

### Using Persona Dolls to ensure inclusive practice

The majority of children in one day nursery are white British, but the population in the area is much more diverse. The manager and staff felt that one useful way to address this balance was through using Persona Dolls, so a black African doll was chosen and the staff received some training. The Persona Doll is now being used to tell stories. In this example the 3- and 4-year-old children have met their doll twice before and already they treat her like a friend. As the practitioner starts today's story he asks them what they remember from the doll's visit to them last week. They remember what made her happy, and that she was sad because in her nursery the other children had not wanted to play with her. They also remembered the ideas they had suggested to help her solve the problem.

## Ensuring well-being

Ferre Laevers is Director of the Research Centre for Experiential Education, based at the Department of Education, Leuven University in Belgium, where he has worked since the 1970s. His work is very well known throughout the UK and in many parts of the world. He frequently speaks at conferences in the UK, explaining his theories of how children learn and, most importantly, what professionals can do to create the right conditions for what he calls "deep level learning" – learning at its most productive.

His work on emotional well-being is very relevant to us as we think about keeping children safe and promoting health and well-being. He sees emotional well-being as having a profound influence on whether or not children are being helped to learn. He has developed observational processes to help practitioners see their settings from the children's perspective and understand the impact on children's learning of their daily routines, learning environments and how adults interact with the children.

His process for assessing the emotional well-being of all the children in a setting is widely used across the UK and elsewhere. It involves making short observations (2–3 minutes) on all the children in the group, looking for certain key signals, such as signs of confidence or lack of it, being relaxed, and a sense of inner peace or signs of discomfort. When well-being is high, as he puts it, the child is "like a fish in water". As the practitioner observes the children, she/he checks them against a five-point scale with a list of statements that describe different levels of well-being, from high to low. The aim is then to take immediate action to support those with low well-being, such as finding out the child's real interests and building on these, or giving the child more personalised adult support.

## Effective practice:
### What do we need to do?

As Linda Pound reminds us, "There is probably no role on earth with greater responsibility for the future of society as well as each individual than practitioners caring for children up to three" (Pound, 2010). This responsibility, shared with parents and principle carers, continues to the end of childhood and schooling. So let us turn now to how we make sure practice in the EYFS is effective.

## Child development

- Get to know each child by finding out about them from the people who know them best – their parents. You will need to find out about what they feel about the child's all-round development, what their child likes to play with and any new skills they are developing. In Chapter 5 there is a list of questions to ask parents, which will be helpful as a starting point.

- Use the information you gather from parents about their children at home, together with what you observe as you play with them, to help tune you into each child. Remember, every child is unique and needs the support that is just right for them, building on their skills, achievements, interests and passions.

## Activity

Find a useful guide to child development, such as *Childcare and Education* by Bruce et al. (2010, pp.53–65). Take one element of child development, such as physical or social development. As you read something about the age of children you are working with, think about some of the children you know. Does what you are reading fit with what you see the children doing? You may find it helpful to carry out this activity with several of your colleagues.

## Inclusive practice

- Help children to respect and value those who are different from themselves by talking with the children about differences in a positive way. Remember that the relationships between the adults in your setting demonstrate to the children how everyone is valued.
- Ensure that the cultural backgrounds of all the children and the wider community are reflected positively in your setting and are demonstrated through displays, resources, leaflets about your setting and policies. Make sure the books and stories for the children give positive images of different cultures, skin tones, disability and gender, as well as a mix of urban and rural settings.
- Make sure that resources for role play, such as kitchen utensils and dressing-up clothes, include those from other cultural heritages. As these may be unusual for the children, make sure the children know how they are used in real life. This is an important aspect of being inclusive – it is not enough to just put resources out. You can do this by getting involved as a play partner.
- Encourage children to develop their understanding of fairness, by being fair and providing opportunities to discuss fairness, for example, using Persona Doll stories.

## Keeping safe

- Ensure you meet all the EYFS statutory requirements that refer to keeping children safe.
- Provide a challenging, creative and stimulating environment for all the children in your care. This means taking safety very seriously by assessing the hazards, then deciding how the risks can be minimised so the interest and challenge for the children remains. Teamwork is vital to ensure everyone adheres to the safety rules.
- Teach children your safety rules as well as how to use tools such as scissors, knives and woodwork tools safely.
- Talk with parents about your risk assessments and procedures for ensuring children are safe. Parents are rightly concerned about the safety of their children, so making sure they are listened to and their concerns are addressed is important.

## Health and well-being

- Take time every few weeks to do a spot check on children's emotional well-being as discussed on page 11. Look around the room and outdoor area two to three times in one session, and note which children seem at ease, energised, confident, happy and secure.
- Talk to other staff about those children whose well-being seems low so that you can plan the best ways of boosting their well-being. This could mean helping them to develop friendships, getting involved in playing alongside them or providing more activities in line with their interests.
- Make sure that the snacks and meals you provide are healthy and children have plenty of time outside.

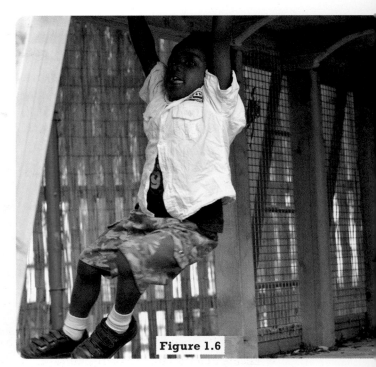

**Figure 1.6**

## Case study: How a Children's Centre meets the Unique Child commitments

At Woodlands Park there is a vibrant, rich and stimulating outdoor area, which provides plenty of opportunities for children to explore nature and the elements, to develop their imagination and creativity and to challenge their physical skills. There is a highly imaginative climbing area with a wooden swing bridge, steps, slide, monkey bars and climbing wall, as well as a water area, taps accessible to the children and a sandpit. There is also an exciting wooded area where children are allowed to climb in one or two of the low trees. This is a truly inclusive environment, ensuring it caters for *all* children. Girls are as active as boys, and children with additional needs are given the support they need to participate in all activities.

Health and safety in the garden is taken very seriously, ensuring that not only is the garden well supervised, but that children know the safety rules and how to look after themselves and others. The staff are positioned so their sightlines are clear, but also so that they can interact with the children, make suggestions to encourage the children's ideas and further their thinking and explorations. Communication between the staff outside is important so that additional support can be given as necessary.

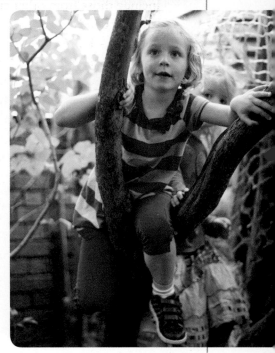

**Figure 1.7** Children know the safety rules about climbing the tree

However, all staff fully understand that their role is not to stand back and supervise, but to interact with the children, supporting them in their explorations and play.

In order to ensure the children are safe, risk assessments are made regularly. There are daily checks on surfaces and potential hazards and staff are always vigilant. A first-aider is always on site. Both staff and the children help to clean up and keep areas tidy.

## Activity

### How does your setting provide for the four commitments of A Unique Child?

Ask the room leaders/supervisors and other staff if each can give you one example of how they feel the setting implements each of the four commitments of A Unique Child. Make a list of their responses. Make sure you get permission from the manager or your supervisor to do this and share it with them. This may provide some valuable contributions to the setting's own self-evaluation. Examples of questions include:

- *A Unique Child*: What do we do here to make sure children are treated as unique and special?
- *Child development*: How does what we provide here show that every aspect of development is equally important?
- *Inclusive practice*: How do we make sure we are inclusive of everyone here? How do we support a child with special needs?
- *Health and well-being*: What do we do here to make sure every child's emotional well-being is supported?

## Chapter summary

Through some examples of effective practice, observations of children and activities to try out, this chapter will have helped you:

➤ understand the EYFS principle A Unique Child and its four commitments, and reflect on your own practice in relation to them
➤ develop your thinking about inclusion and how to ensure your practice is inclusive
➤ learn about what two experts have to say about inclusion and well-being.

# Further reading and references

Brown, B. (1999) *Unlearning Discrimination in the Early Years*, Trentham Books Ltd, Stoke-on-Trent

Brown, B. (2008) *Equality in Action: A Way Forward with Persona Dolls*, Trentham Books Ltd, Stoke-on-Trent

Bruce, T., Meggitt, C. and Grenier, J. (2010) *Childcare and Education*, Hodder Education, London

Hutchin, V. (2003) *Observing and Assessing for the Foundation Stage Profile*, Hodder Education, London

Laevers, F. (2000) 'Forward to basics! Deep-level-learning and the Experiential Approach', *Early Years*, Vol. 20, No. 2

Lindon J. (1999) *Too Safe for their Own Good*, National Early Years Network, London

Pound, L. (2010) *Contemporary Thinking and Theorists*, Practical Pre-school Books, MA Education Ltd, London

## Useful websites

Early Years national policy documents for England and other useful information for practitioners and parents can be found at: www.foundationyears.org.uk

Persona Doll Training: www.persona-doll-training.org

# Chapter 2

# Positive Relationships

## In this chapter we will be looking at:

➤ the commitments for Positive Relationships, paying particular attention to the key person

➤ observations of children as they learn and develop and how positive relationships within their settings have helped them

➤ what research by some key experts is telling us about the importance of positive relationships and the role of the key person

➤ what we do to ensure our practice is effective, with a case study on how one setting has developed the role of the key person.

## Introduction

Four 3-year-olds are playing at the dough table. Each has a large ball of warm, soft, malleable dough that they have just made. They are squishing, pulling or kneading their pieces. A fifth child comes along and stands near the table watching. He is a new child and does not yet know the other children well. He looks a little upset but says nothing. His key person arrives at the table to support him. She provides a chair for him, knowing he is not yet ready to sit down, but so it will be there for him when he is ready. She asks the others kindly if they will share some of their dough with him. First one child pulls off a piece of dough and gives it to him, then the others follow. How did the children learn to be so inclusive? What is a key person and how did she help him? This chapter answers these questions.

Positive relationships are at the very centre of enabling children to learn. From the base of sensitive, warm, reciprocal relationships within the family, babies and young children begin to develop the self-confidence to branch out, explore their environment, become involved in new experiences and form new relationships outside the immediate circle of family. Once they begin to attend an early years setting or a childminder, the positive relationships between practitioners and the children and families are essential for the children to continue their developmental journey without interruption. Children, just like adults, cannot develop and learn when they feel unhappy, emotionally insecure or anxious: close, supportive relationships make all the difference, right through the EYFS years, into Key Stage 1 and beyond.

## The EYFS principle, Positive Relationships, tells us:

*"Children learn to be strong and independent through positive relationships."*

(EYFS, 2012)

'Positive Relationships' is the second of the four themes of the EYFS and is closely linked to the other three, especially the first theme of 'A Unique Child'. As we will see in this chapter, the 'key person' is central in building these positive relationships. The assignment of a key person to every child is a *requirement* in all settings,

*"to help ensure that every child's care is tailored to meet their individual needs... help the child become familiar with the setting, offer a settled relationship and build a relationship with their parents".*

(EYFS Framework, 2012)

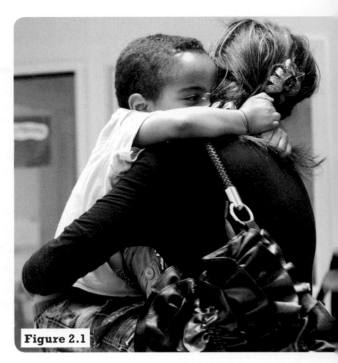

Figure 2.1

## What is this theme about?

There are four supporting commitments for the theme of Positive Relationships. They help us to see what we need to do to enable children to feel at ease, happy and develop as confident and independent learners.

The supporting commitments within Positive Relationships are:
- Respecting each other
- Parents as partners
- Supporting learning
- Key person

## Respecting each other

*"Every interaction is based on caring professional relationships and respectful acknowledgement of the feelings of children and their families."*

(EYFS card 2.1)

A truly respectful environment is one where everyone – children and adults – feels valued and fully included. Respect for each other is an important part of inclusive practice, as discussed in the last chapter. In an inclusive setting everyone is welcomed and accepted for who they are, their cultures and beliefs are acknowledged, respected and celebrated, and no one suffers discrimination. In this respectful community we are all learners – not just the children – and part of what we are learning is how to respect others' points of view, even when they are very different from our own. As Helen Bromley says, "It is easy to be blinded by difference and to see it as a barrier to effective communication... valuing what binds us together may yet be the most effective way to build partnerships based on empathy and trust" (Bromley, 2011).

Creating an inclusive environment for the children and their families helps the children learn to respect and value others. Most of all it helps them to know that they really matter. Children come to understand about other people's feelings by watching how others respond, not only to themselves but to others too. They notice how different people may respond to the same event in a different way to themselves. They learn about empathy and often need help to express their feelings in acceptable ways. We all have very strong feelings from time to time, and managing these is a skill we continue to develop throughout life. For most children, the first time they are with other children outside the immediate circle of family and family friends for an extended period of time is when they begin attending a setting or a childminder.

## Valuing ourselves and valuing our colleagues

To work as an effective team all team members need to develop trust in and respect for each other. We may not agree with the views of every team member or with some parents' views, but this should not affect our respect for them as people. As the EYFS 2008 says, "If you value and respect yourself, you will do the same for others."

# Parents as partners

"Parents are children's first and most enduring educators. When parents and practitioners work together in early years settings, the results have a positive impact on children's development and learning."

(EYFS card 2.2)

In the early years positive relationships with parents have always been considered fundamental: for parents to hand over charge of their child to the setting depends on them feeling that this is the right place for their child. Over the past few years the importance of a true partnership with parents has been increasingly emphasised, not just in the early years but throughout the school years. In 2011 the Tickell Review of the EYFS prioritised partnership with parents as an area that needs further development nationally. In this book we have devoted a whole chapter to it – see Chapter 5 to find out more.

# Supporting learning

"Warm, trusting relationships with knowledgeable adults support children's learning more effectively than any amount of resources."

(EYFS card 2.3)

Our relationships with children are the key resource for learning. SPEEL, a research project on early learning for 3- to 5-year-olds reported in 2002 that "all previous research and evaluation projects conducted in the UK and internationally point conclusively to the quality of the interaction between practitioners and children in the three–five years age range as critical to the... long-term successful outcomes of children's early learning." As an early years adviser, if I want to know how effective the practice is in a setting I first look at the relationships and interaction between the staff and the children. Other things do matter as well of course, but this is the key.

So what do we need to do to support learning? Begin by taking time to find out about the children with whom you are going to be working: what are their passions, worries and concerns? What are they already able to do? How confident are they feeling about attending your setting? This means finding out from parents/carers and listening to and observing the children themselves. We often refer to how we support children's learning as our 'pedagogy'. It includes the attentiveness and care we give to the children, how we interact with them as well as what we might call 'teaching'. It also includes the learning environment we provide and how this is used to support learning. The case study below gives an example of how the pedagogy of effective practitioners supports learning.

## Case study: **Katie, age 4**

Katie only feels at ease when she knows what to expect each day; for example, when her key person greets her every day she takes her to see the visual timetable – a display along the wall into the group room which provides a timeline of the day through photographs of the children at play: in small group time, snack time and lunchtime, and being collected at the end of the day. As Katie is one of the children in the photographs, being able to identify herself is additional support for her. Not only has this helped her separate from her mother every day, but it has also helped new children settle in and all the children to understand the passage of time. This has helped the setting to be more inclusive.

## Activity

Make a timeline with photographs of the children taken at different key times of day, such as arriving, saying goodbye to parents, playing inside and outside, with some of the activities available, including snack, story time, and so on. Display this along the wall where children can touch and refer to it, with captions explaining the time of day. It is a good idea to laminate it!

## Key person

*"A key person has special responsibilities for working with a small number of children, giving them reassurance to feel safe and cared for and building relationships with their parents."*

(EYFS card 2.4)

## Attachment

Babies are completely dependent for everything on their principle carers, which usually begins with parents, especially the mother. As they try to make sense of the way their world works it is the reciprocal relationships and the unconditional love and care they receive that makes this possible. They soon become "attached" to their main carer in a special way, and from about 6 months old the bond is so strong that they become very wary, if not frightened of being left with anyone to whom they are not emotionally attached. They may become inconsolable if they do not know the person looking after them well enough. The baby or child feels understandably frightened about what is happening to them and for how long, especially when their language development is at an early stage.

Attachment is a major aspect of early childhood development that needs to be taken very seriously. It is like an invisible thread linking the baby and young child to the significant adults in his or her life. If the attachment is not secure or is abruptly broken by circumstances it is very likely to cause some difficulties in later life. Forming secure attachments is vital to children's emotional development, and it is from these strong emotional bonds that they gain the security, confidence and resilience to become independent and form positive relationships with others. Secure attachments support their cognitive development in two ways. First, no one can learn when they feel frightened and unhappy, and second, the positive feedback that the baby receives from their caregiver provides the confidence to try new things.

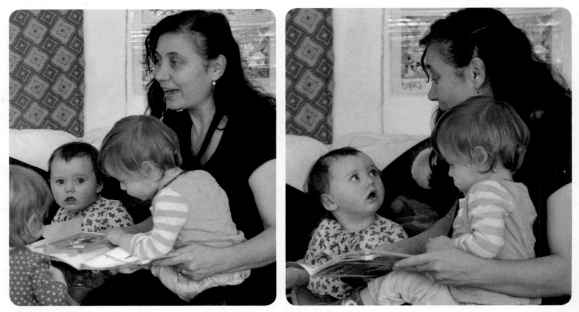

**Figure 2.2** This baby is feeling anxious at seeing a stranger, but the problem is soon resolved by her key person.

There are a number of important qualities that the adult brings to enable the baby/child to feel secure and make secure attachments, from which they gain in confidence and grow from being dependent emotionally to being independent. These are:

- care and love
- consistency
- predictability
- dependability
- and, most importantly, being *emotionally there* for the child when he or she needs it most.

Babies and young children do not only form attachments with their parents or principle caregivers; attachments will be formed with other familiar adults who provide all of these qualities, and this is likely to be the key person in the setting.

## What is a key person?

The key person is a designated person who takes on a very special responsibility for individual children in the setting while those on whom the child depends are not there. The concept of a key person was already quite established as a statutory requirement in England in 2008, because ensuring children's emotional security is so important. It is statutory throughout the EYFS age range because smooth transition from home to setting or school is so important to children's learning. Peter Elfer and colleagues describe the key person's role in this way:

*"The key person makes sure that, within the day-to-day demands of a nursery each child feels individual, cherished and thought about by someone in particular while they are away from home."*

(Elfer *et al.*, 2002, p.18)

The key person approach in all settings makes a big difference to children and parents when it is well planned and thoughtfully implemented. The key person finds out all about the child or baby, helps them to settle in when they first start, and works out with the parents the individual settling-in procedures that will best suit their child. Of course, if you are a childminder, you are the key person to all the children in your care. In a nursery or school setting, the key person forms the strongest relationship between the setting, child and family.

## What are the expectations?

The expectations of the key person role are high: the key person is not only the one in whose hands the parent leaves the child every day, but, ideally, is the person who is there to give feedback at the end of the day on how it went. As the key person, you are the one the parent talks to if there are any concerns or worries, and the person responsible for intimate care such as nappy changing or toileting, and the one available if the child is upset. Because you build such a close relationship with the child, he or she turns to you for comfort. This is not the same attachment as the children have to their close family, but you are nevertheless the most important person to the child in the setting.

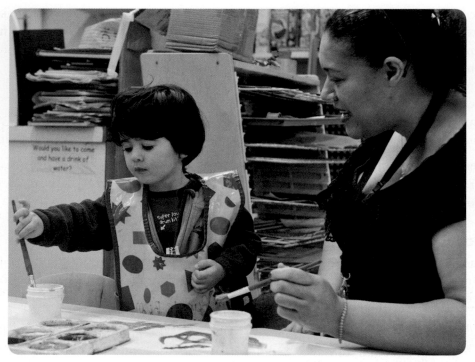

**Figure 2.3** A new child is supported to get involved in an activity by his key person

All of this is a big responsibility, but the rewards of being that person who is so significant in the child's life brings with it the joy that a close, caring relationship brings, seeing the child develop and playing a part in their learning. Your responsibilities will include observing the child and keeping records up to date. To get the key person approach working well is about offering consistent, dependable and nurturing support for the child, making them feel cared about, respected and valued. This is an essential component of inclusive practice. It requires good management as well as a good level of understanding of the role by all involved. We look at these issues in the Effective practice section of this chapter.

## Looking at children:
## What do we see?

### Louis, age 3 years 2 months

Louis has been in the nursery school for two months. His parents have told his key person that his big passion at present is trains, particularly Thomas the Tank Engine and friends, so during his first few days his key person made sure the train track was out and that he knew where to find it and how to get it out. His key person and the staff team in his group are gradually introducing him to the wide range of experiences on offer to support his learning. Today he has shown some interest in the computer, watching others use it. A member of staff who is nearby sees this and introduces him to the mouse and the paint program the others were using to draw. The practitioner helps him to control the mouse. He begins to make marks, showing his delight and pleasure at the marks he is making. He looked at the print of his first drawing and said in a very quiet voice, "I made a choo Thomas." After this and before each drawing, he told the practitioner what he was going to draw: "It's choo Thomas" or "I want a Diesel." When she asked him which he liked best, Thomas or Diesel, his response was: "Diesel faster!"

## What have we found out?

The practitioner's awareness of Louis's interest in trains has enabled her to provide the sensitive support Louis needs to explore something new to him. She listens carefully to what he is saying in a very quiet voice and uses this to talk with him about it, extending the conversation. Her focused attention and positive relationship with him gives him the opportunity to gain in confidence and skill in using the mouse and in expressing himself.

## Veronica, age 8 months

Veronica's key person made this observation as she sat near her:

*"This is Veronica's third day in nursery and the first time her mother has left her for any length of time. Her mother says goodbye to her and Veronica smiles back. She sits very close to her key person, feeling and mouthing some of the baby toys which are within reach, listening to the noises around, turning herself around to see when others enter the room. She is vocalising contentedly. An older child comes over and plays with some of the toys, chatting about what she is doing. Veronica watches her then shuffles on her bottom to get a bit nearer. The older child gives her one of the toys which Veronica takes, putting it in her mouth."*

## What have we found out?

Veronica appears relaxed and contented on her third day in the nursery, the first time her mother has left her. She seems curious about the sounds she hears as well as what she can see and reach, exploring these using her senses. She is interested in watching the older child and confident and curious enough to approach her. The key person nearby is helping her to feel confident.

## What the experts say
### Attachment and relationships

The theory of attachment was based on the work of Dr John Bowlby, who began his research in the 1950s. He was interested in what happens to children when they are separated from their principle caregivers. His research concluded that insecure attachments in infancy are likely to have a negative impact on behaviour in later childhood and throughout life. His work has had considerable impact on later research and on professionals working in social care, health and early childhood.

In 2007 a beautifully illustrated and very useful short booklet, edited by John Oates at the Open University was published. It brings together seven experts on attachment and young children's learning and development from around the world. Each of the experts has written a page summarising simply some research on attachment. The booklet is called *Attachment Relationships* and is part of a series called 'Early Childhood in Focus'. It is available on the internet. The book opens with the following statement:

*"In recent years, an extensive body of research has been accumulating, showing that the early care environment has a major role in a child's development... Central to these effects is the quality of the attachment bonds that a child forms with the persons who provide care, such as parents, other members of the family or community, or professional carers."*

(Oates, 2007, vii)

## The key person role

The idea of attachment helps us to understand how separation from the main caregivers must feel to the child, and to recognise the need for strong personal, supportive relationships between practitioners and children developed through the key person approach.

In 2002, several years before the EYFS became the statutory framework, Peter Elfer from the Early Childhood Studies Department at Roehampton University introduced the key person as a requirement when he wrote a very useful book with Elinor Goldschmied and Dorothy Selleck entitled *Key Persons in the Nursery*. In the book they describe the key person approach as "a way of working in nurseries in which the whole focus of the organisation is aimed at enabling and supporting close attachments between individual children and individual nursery staff" (Elfer et al, 2005). They go on to explain that this is in no way replacing the attachment of the parent, but is a partnership with the parent: "... it gives the parents the chance to liaise with someone else who is fully committed and familiar with their baby". In contrast to this is what Julian Grenier calls "the impersonal care" that tended to take place in "impersonal nurseries", where "anyone can change nappies at a time which is convenient to the organisation. Children may be processed across the nappy changing table like tins of beans travelling along the checkout at a supermarket" (EYFS, 2008). Hopefully this poor practice no longer exists.

## Effective practice:
### What do we need to do?

## Respecting each other

### Building respectful relationships and team spirit

- Create an ethos of respect and a respectful environment by making sure everyone is welcomed and their views and feelings can be expressed. Being respectful helps others to be respectful too.
- Celebrate the similarities as well as differences among the staff team, the parents and the children.
- Ensure that no one feels excluded. Demonstrate the care and concern you have for others by being an attentive listener. This is particularly important for parents – their views may not always coincide with yours, but they need to be given time to express them and have a conversation with you about them – even if sometimes you agree to differ. If you need support in this be sure to talk to your line manager or mentor.

- Build a team spirit by keeping in mind the key objective of an early years setting: to provide the best for the child. Ensuring everyone is clear about their roles and responsibilities will help all to feel valued.
- Think about how your setting feels from the child's perspective. Is it welcoming, enjoyable and supportive?

### Activity

Reflect on the routines and procedures in your setting, for example, taking turns on the outdoor equipment. Are the procedures clear to the children? If some of the routines and procedures cause friction or unhappiness, what can be done to improve the situation? Think about what would help – for example, for 2–5-year-olds, having a clipboard where children can write their names or make a mark to show they want a turn on the bikes. Talk to the children about it. Take some photographs to help children understand how the turn-taking process works. With the children put these into a sequence and display it so they can refer to it.

### Helping children develop respect, manage feelings and build friendships

- Help children learn to respect others by showing your genuine respect for others, being open and accepting, showing respect for the environment and the local community.
- Support young children to develop friendships by getting involved in play alongside them. Pairing the child up with another child who is showing similar interests or tends to play in a similar way can be very helpful.
- Talk about feelings. This is important in nurturing children's respect and empathy. Children, like adults, have very strong feelings from time to time, so help them understand these and find appropriate ways of expressing them. A calm, supportive environment helps.
- Help children manage their feelings by using some of the excellent storybooks for young children about feelings.
- A very useful strategy for promoting empathy, helping children to recognise similarities and differences between themselves and others and respect difference is to use Persona Dolls.

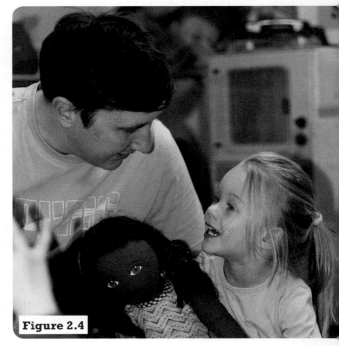
**Figure 2.4**

#### Persona Dolls

Persona dolls are special dolls, suitable for children age 3 years and up, that are used to tell stories with a purpose. They provide a practical, effective way to raise issues of fairness and equality with young children and encourage them to develop empathy and value difference. The dolls and their stories need to reflect diversity. In settings where all the children are white British, for example, a Persona Doll from a different ethnic background can 'tell' stories that highlight lifestyle similarities and differences. Practitioners create a personality and a family and cultural background for the dolls, just as if they were real children. Once their 'personas' have been created, the practitioner sits the doll on his/her lap to 'tell' the doll's stories. The children are given the time and space to help solve the problems the dolls encounter. The children easily get into the magic of storytelling, treat the dolls as real people, identify with them and care about what happens to them. They enthusiastically contribute their ideas, talk about their personal experiences and readily respond to the problems posed.

To keep the dolls' lives as real as possible and to avoid presenting them as victims, practitioners also tell stories about happy events, such as going to a party. At other times the stories address issues of unfairness. Perhaps a doll is called a hurtful name because of her/his skin colour or disability. A boy doll may tell a story about the girls in 'his setting' not letting him play with dolls, or a girl doll's story may be about the boys excluding her from the construction area.

## Activity

Find out more about Persona Dolls and discuss this approach with your colleagues or your team. Try creating a persona for a doll and write it down – once a doll has a persona and a background, it can be added to, but the basic facts such as the family background cannot be changed, just like in real life! Get a colleague to help you devise a story on an issue about fairness relevant to your setting. Then try a Persona Doll session with a small group of children who you know well. If you have never tried telling a story, try a traditional tale with story props first to a very small group. This will help you to build confidence. See the website references at the end of the chapter.

## Supporting learning

- Find out and follow children's interests. This is the best starting point for extending learning.
- Talk to parents/carers informally every day so that you can update each other on what the child is doing in your setting and at home.
- Observe and listen carefully to the children before you get involved, showing your interest in what the children have chosen to do.
- Plan time to be involved in children's self-initiated play. When children are involved in imaginative play and role play, get involved as a "play partner".
- Be flexible in the adult-led activities so that you can accommodate the children's particular interests. Adult-led activities are best when they come from the children's interests, so that the new learning you are introducing is relevant to them.
- Ask the children open-ended questions so they have plenty of time to think and talk, come up with their own ideas and solve problems. Speculating with the children can help: "I wonder what would happen if..."
- Bring an element of surprise into the familiar activities and experiences you provide, as this can often prompt children to think in a new way – for example, reading a familiar story slightly wrong or changing some key word in songs. Sharing a joke with a child because you said the wrong word can be a great way to get children thinking.

### What is it like for a child here?

Choose a child to observe, for example, a child who is generally very quiet with both other children and adults. Watch the child at play for a few minutes, then return to watch again after half an hour or so. Have you found out anything new you did not know before about the child's interests or how the child got involved in an activity? Is there anything more that could be done to make the child feel more fully involved, for example, helped to play with others by a member of staff or the key person being nearby? Share your observation with your manager or room leader.

## Key person

To establish the key person approach effectively requires careful planning, good team work and time for regular reviews to ensure it is working well for everyone – child, family and staff. Here are some of the dilemmas of the key person approach that may arise, and the solutions:

- *Dilemma*: How can the key person *always* be on hand for the child? In day care settings staff are on shifts and some staff may be part-time. When a setting is open all year round, staff need to take their holidays when their key children are still attending.
  *Solution*: Organise the staff in pairs to be "co-key persons" for each other's key group, so that the co-key person is available when the key person is not there. Make sure information is passed on as necessary at handover times and the children and parents are aware of whom to go to when the key person is not present.

- *Dilemma*: How can the key person keep track of all her/his key children in a large, open-plan setting for children age 3 upwards?
  *Solution*: Effective team work helps, making sure all staff know which children are in which key group. Organise group times so that each key person is with just their key children. Make sure there is time to discuss the children at planning meetings and, where possible, at a short feedback session at the end of the day.

- *Dilemma*: What if parents are concerned that their child's strong relationship with his or her key person will affect his or her own relationship with their child?
  *Solution*: Reassure parents that the key person relationship can never replace them – they are the most important people to the child. Even though you are very special to the child, your role is as a professional.

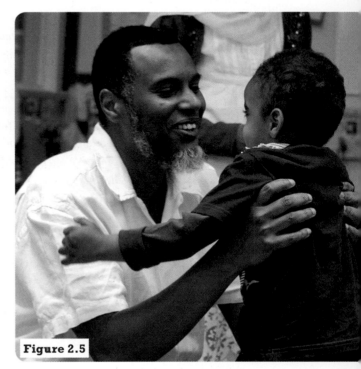

**Figure 2.5**

Parents can be very anxious about leaving their child in the care of someone else. Feedback to parents at the end of the day is important.

■ *Dilemma*: If there are a large number of children in each key group, how can the observations be kept up to date, particularly in a large, open-plan setting?

*Solution*: Every staff member can contribute to each child's record, but the key person is responsible for collating them, sharing them with parents and thinking about the next steps for her/his key children.

## Case study: The key person approach at Woodlands Park Children's Centre

Woodlands Park is a large, maintained nursery school and Children's Centre with all-year-round provision for children from 7 months to 5 years. Some of the children are part-time and term-time only and some stay all day, all year round. The role of the key person is taken very seriously, and the strong, friendly, respectful and positive relationships between the children, staff and parents are tangible to any visitor. Of the 12 staff working with the under-3s, seven of them take on the role of key person. In my discussion with the Under Threes Coordinator, Jenny, she told me:

*"When the children see the trusting relationship between us and their parents they feel they can trust us too. For the child the key person is their special person at nursery. It is really important that the key person takes care of the child through the intimate times such as nappy changing, sleep and meal times. This is when they really need someone who is special to them. We also have a key group time we call 'island time' just before lunch where the children are grouped with their key person. They all know, babies and toddlers included, where their island time space is and who they will be with. It is an important time for them and is like a family group as each key person has children from babies to three years in their group."*

For the parents, the key person is their key point of contact.

*"We are not stepping into parents' shoes. We know we need to be sensitive when we give feedback at the end of the day so that working parents don't feel they have missed out, we ensure they hear about what the child has been doing. We often provide support to parents too as they can feel quite isolated when they are working. They may not know many other parents, so we can help by telling them who their child is playing with at nursery. We often have social events too such as the international evenings where everyone brings some food. Parents really welcome these occasions."*

Every child also has a co-key person as well as their key person. The co-key person can take responsibility for a child when the key person is not available. This helps ensure consistency for the child.

*"We introduce the 'co-key person' to the child gradually at first so that they know their key person best first. They may start to get to know their co-key person by sitting next to her at lunch time for instance."*

*"Team work is the key to success. Everyone knows who each key person and co-key person is responsible for. If anyone is in need of some support – perhaps a child is not well or a little unhappy one day, then we help each other out. The support staff are always there to help too."*

Most importantly, if someone less experienced is unsure what to say to a parent, for example, they know that they can talk it through with another staff member.

## Chapter summary

This chapter will have helped you:
➤ understand the EYFS principle Positive Relationships
➤ find out why attachment and the key person role are so important from some experts in the field
➤ reflect on your setting's practice in relation to the key person role and see how one setting is ensuring the key person role and building positive relationships is at the heart of their practice.

## Further reading and references

Bromley, H, 'Accepted Practice', *Nursery World*, 18–31 October 2011, pp.24–5

Elfer, P., Goldschmied, E. and Selleck, D. (2005) *Key Persons in the Nursery: Building Relationships for Quality Provision*, David Fulton Publishers Ltd, London

Grenier, J. (2008) quoted in Early Years Foundation Stage, 2008: www.foundationyears.org.uk

Oates, J., (2007) *Attachment Relationships*, Early Childhood in Focus 1, M. Woodhead and J. Oates (eds.), The Open University, Milton Keynes. The whole series of booklets are downloadable at: www.bernardvanleer.org/English/Home/Our-publications/Browse_by_series.html?ps_page=1&getSeries=3

### Useful websites

Persona Doll Training: www.persona-doll-training.org

# Chapter 3

# Enabling Environments

## In this chapter we will be looking at:

➤ the commitments for Enabling Environments, paying particular attention to Observation, assessment and planning and The learning environment

➤ children learning and developing in an enabling, inclusive environment

➤ some key research on observing and listening to children and the importance of outdoor learning

➤ what we do to ensure our practice is effective in supporting learning, with a case study on how some settings have developed their learning environments.

## Introduction

Davi, who is 4 years old, is new to learning English. Today he was very involved in playing with water and some guttering placed sloping from the fence to the water tray on the ground. He was deeply involved, going to the nearby tap to fill buckets with water and pouring it down the guttering. He also poured the water from one bucket to another and straight from the bucket onto the ground. He watched intently as the water filled the bucket and spilled over, running down the plughole in the sink, and said, "Going down here!" He laughed when Advan let a dinosaur go down the guttering and it splashed into the water tray at the bottom. When Advan said, "Splash", Davi repeated the word "splash" delightedly.

This experience has been an *enabling* one for Davi, helping him to explore the properties and momentum of flowing water and to be involved with others. It is also helping his development in English. The environment with its accessible resources encouraged him to explore the flow of the water and there are also positive relationships supporting him: a practitioner, who observed the play, and another child who is playing alongside him. Both support his learning and development and enable him to explore, learn about the properties of water and communicate in a new language.

## The EYFS principle, Enabling Environments, tells us:

"Children learn and develop well in enabling environments, in which their experiences respond to their individual needs and there is a strong partnership between practitioners and parents and/or carers."

(EYFS Statutory Framework, 2012)

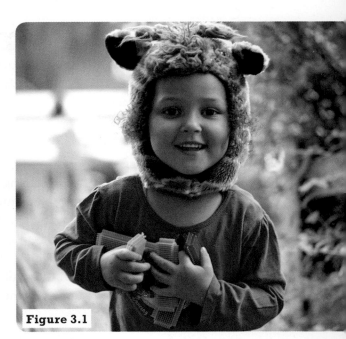

**Figure 3.1**

The third principle of the EYFS is all about providing children with Enabling Environments. The word "enable" means to make possible or facilitate, so an enabling environment for young children is one where children's learning and development are made possible. It is a useful word that is full of action. The observation of Davi's play described on the previous page demonstrates an enabling environment in action. We can see how an enabling environment is closely linked with the first two principles of A Unique Child and Positive Relationships as well as the fourth principle of Learning and Development.

## What is this theme about?

The principle is not just about the physical environment inside and outdoors. The effective environment caters for the varied ways in which children learn. Children are encouraged to be creative and their imaginations are fired up. They are motivated to explore, discover things that are new to them and try out new ways of doing things. And central to all of this is what you, the practitioners, do to support children to become resilient, resourceful learners, full of energy, curiosity and with a zest to find out more.

The four supporting commitments demonstrate the breadth covered by the theme of Enabling Environments:

■ Observation, assessment and planning
■ Supporting every child
■ The learning environment
■ The wider context.

# Observation, assessment and planning

*"Babies and young children are individuals first, each with a unique profile of abilities. Schedules and routines should flow with the child's needs. All planning starts with observing children in order to understand and consider their current interests, development and learning."*

(EYFS card 3.1)

## Observing

You might think that under the heading of Enabling Environments is an odd place to find out about observation, assessment and planning in the EYFS. But creating the best environment for the children requires practitioners to find out about them from observing them and then, from what has been seen, planning ways to inspire them further, foster their interests and engage them in discovering and learning more. This ensures that your provision for children's learning is not a hit-and-miss affair, but fully tailored to their needs. As the Effective Practice section of the 2008 EYFS on observation, assessment and planning puts it:

*"Without observation, overall planning would be simply based on what we felt was important, fun or interesting (or all three) but it might not meet the needs of children in our care."*

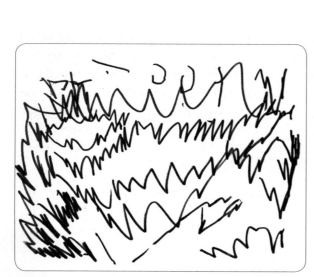

**Figure 3.2** Charlie's writing: "It just says macaroni" – Charlie, age 4

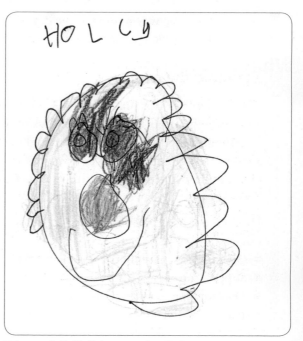

**Figure 3.3** Holly's portrait – Holly, age 4

Observation, assessment and planning work in a continuous cycle:

- It starts with *observing* the children. Observing means watching and listening. This is the evidence-gathering stage in the cycle.
- Next comes the *assessment* part of the cycle. Asking questions can help with making assessments – for example, from our knowledge of child development, what are we finding out about *what* and *how* the child appears to be learning? What skills are being developed?
- The next part of the cycle is the *planning*: what can we do as a result of what we found out? What play possibilities and opportunities should we provide next and how should practitioners be involved?
- The final stage is *making it happen*: implementing the plans and motivating the children to participate by making sure the environment and the learning experiences are appealing and well planned.

Chapter 16 spells out each step of the cycle in detail.

## Involving parents and children

Within the evidence-gathering stage in the cycle is information you have gathered from talking with parents and any other professionals who may be involved. An important part of the evidence gathered about a child's learning comes from parents. This means time needs to be made to ensure there are frequent conversations about what the child is doing at home. At the assessment stage you will also need to include parents' views and the child's views too. Can you find an effective way to ensure the children's views are included? Even the youngest? For more information, look at the section later in this chapter on what the experts say.

## Planning the overview

Planning based on observations is the most important aspect of planning. It guides what will be provided and how on a daily basis, but it *depends on* having a longer-term view of planning. I call this planning the overview. It is dependent on knowing all about child development and what you want the children to be learning and developing in the long term, over the whole of the time they are with you. This is how you will ensure that you are covering all the areas of learning of the EYFS and the different aspects within it. It provides a general overview of how you make it happen, including the continuous provision available to the children at all times and, in general terms, how practitioners support play as well as adult-led activities.

Many settings use the Development Matters guidance as their long-term planning overview. However, your own setting's planning overview provides the basis for the all-important regular evaluation of the setting, helping you to ensure you are providing children with a breadth of experiences through the play environment you create and the activities and opportunities you make available. So the overview for your own setting is also important.

## Oh no, not record keeping!

Most practitioners would agree that one of the most interesting aspects of working with young children is working out how you can best support their learning. This depends on observation and is vital in ensuring you meet the needs of *every* child. When the EYFS was reviewed in 2011 some concern was expressed about the requirement to carry out observations, taking practitioners away from interacting with the children. But most observation is carried out *as* you interact with the children, watching, listening and responding to them. Only a new development that seems significant for the child needs to be written down. The only point of observing children is to put the evidence gathered to good use! Observations are not for storing in folders and cupboards, but to *inform your planning.* For this reason it has remained a statutory requirement to observe children:

*"Ongoing assessment (also known as formative assessment) is an integral part of the learning and development process."*

(Statutory Framework, 2012)

This requirement continues right through to the end of the EYFS when the statutory assessment for the EYFS Profile is made.

## Supporting every child

*"The environment supports every child's learning through planned experiences and activities that are challenging but achievable."*

(EYFS card 3.2)

This commitment chimes well with the principles of A Unique Child and Positive Relationships, but the difference is the emphasis on how the environment we set up supports children's learning and development. How can we make sure it supports *every* child? What are we doing to support children who have special needs? What about children who are showing special abilities and talents? What about the quiet and shy children and the boisterous, noisy and active children? To answer these questions we need to be vigilant and review and reflect on what we are providing and how the children are responding. When the environment and what we plan to do within it is right then every child feels at ease and is fully engaged. As Ferre Laevers so aptly put it, the child should be "like a fish in water".

## The learning environment

*"A rich and varied environment supports children's learning and development. It gives them the confidence to explore and learn in secure and safe, yet challenging, indoor and outdoor spaces."*

(EYFS card 3.3)

### What should the environment do?

The learning environment is not just about the physical environment inside and outdoors. It also includes the emotional environment. The right emotional environment ensures children feel safe and secure through positive, consistent and supportive relationships. This gives children the confidence to explore and make use of the physical environment.

Both the environment indoors and the environment outdoors should:
■ provoke children to be thoughtful
■ foster curiosity
■ motivate children to discover and explore for themselves
■ stir the imagination and encourage creativity
■ inspire a sense of wonder and delight.

Carefully planned, the environment becomes a powerful teacher. As the Effective Practice section in the 2008 EYFS states: "To foster progress, settings should create an environment that achieves a balance between providing enough of the familiar to reassure while presenting enough of the new to stimulate and extend."

### Safety first

The spaces provided inside and out must be safe, secure, free from hazards and clean. This is a daily priority. Keeping spaces and resources fresh and tidy can make all the difference between children being able to learn from them or not. It also makes us all feel better! And it means that the environment will be treated with pride and respect by the children and the adults.

## Accessibility of resources

Resources should be easily accessible to the children. They need to be the resources that are appropriate to the children's ages and stages of development and feed their particular interests. It is not a question of making everything accessible all the time, but thinking about what is right for now and then giving children the go-ahead to choose. Teamwork is important: all members of the team need to work to the same policy. Children need to know the rules about choosing and tidying away.

## Tidying away

Of course with younger children, mobile babies and toddlers in particular, the resources are likely to be transported about in all sorts of ways, and sometimes just dropped on the floor. Boxes of resources can be tipped out deliberately and with delight to learn about the effect! This is all part of exploration and is crucial to children's learning about how materials work, but once the exploration is over, tidying up and encouraging the children to be involved is also important. For pack-away settings, the organisation around tidying and setting up each day has to be meticulous. Those not working in a pack-away setting can learn a great deal about how to keep things tidy and carefully stored from how pack-away settings do it.

Although the children will not necessarily be interested in tidying, when you know the children well you can tap into this to find the best way they might help. For example, the children who love to fill the dressing-up bags with all sorts of interesting things that they then carry with them everywhere can help by showing you where they have put things, and then help to sort them. Tidying is usually a very good mathematical experience, as children categorise, sort and count things back in the boxes.

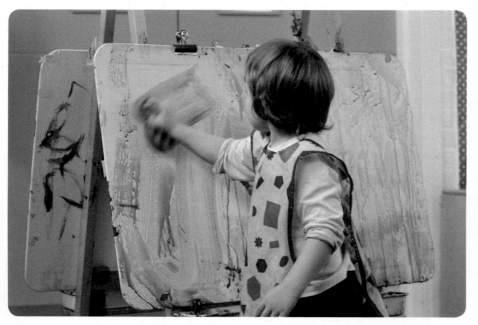

**Figure 3.4** Asking children to help tidy up in line with their particular interests means it is more likely to work!

## A vibrant outdoor environment

Many children in the UK spend far too little time experiencing the outdoor world, even in rural areas. Yet we know that experiencing fresh air, the weather and the richness of nature is fundamental to their learning right from babyhood. Have you noticed how children want to be outside more than they want to be in? If there is not a free flow between the inside areas and the outdoors, they wait for the door to be opened and then burst through with great enthusiasm. Why? As Jan White, an expert on creating stimulating outdoor learning environments, says, "The real contact with the elements, seasons, sensations and environments ... and the daily change, uncertainty, surprise and excitement all contribute to the desire young children have to be outside" (White, 2009).

Our concerns should not be about the boisterous nature of those champing at the bit to get outside, but about those children who find outdoors daunting because they lack confidence. We need to make sure there are quiet spaces for them outside and adults who are available to encourage their explorations by getting alongside them.

The great thing about the outdoors is that it is so very different from being inside. Children are able to engage physically with the elements in a way they cannot do inside. Not every outdoor environment is full of nature. However, there is a lot that can be done quite easily to ensure that nature is introduced, by experiencing the weather and introducing planters and natural materials such as logs, a digging patch and safe but challenging climbing equipment. Many early years settings in both urban and rural settings are part of the Forest School Movement. There is more information about Forest Schools in Chapter 14.

## Reviewing your outdoor provision

Consider the following questions and observe to find out the answers.

1 Are there quiet spaces for children to think and wonder, as well as things to climb and areas to be active and boisterous?

2 What do the children spend most time doing outside? How can it be extended?

3 When you observe children playing outside, how many areas of learning can you see when you analyse your observation? Are there differences between what the boys do and what the girls do?

4 Do you think some children are missing out on the breadth of experiences

# The wider context

*"Working in partnership with other settings, other professionals and with individuals and groups in the community supports children's development and progress ..."*

(EYFS card 3.4)

The final commitment under Enabling Environments is all about developing partnerships with other agencies and with the wider local community. The Tickell Review of the EYFS in 2011 flagged up partnership between professionals to support children and families as an area for development nationally, particularly where a child may need additional support. There are some very good models of practice already and the development of Children's Centres has been important in building strong partnerships between professionals and with parents. In many settings the key person is involved in writing the IEP (Individual Education Plan) with the SENCO and other professionals. The Every Child a Talker programme (see Chapter 10) has been very useful in ensuring that speech and language therapists work more closely with early years practitioners and parents to support children's language development.

The Common Assessment Framework (CAF) was developed to ensure all professionals involved with a child needing additional support work together.

*"The CAF is a shared assessment and planning framework for use across all children's services and all local areas in England. It aims to help the early identification of children's additional needs and promote co-ordinated service provision to meet them."*

(Children's Workforce Development Council website – www.cwdcouncil.org.uk)

# Looking at children:
## What do we see?

### William, age 19 months

William uses the rich learning environment extremely well to explore what takes his interest. He seems confident in the mixed age group setting with children from babies to 3 years. In this observation he is in the home corner, initially alone. He discovers newly introduced resources, including some real vegetables and fruit in a basket.

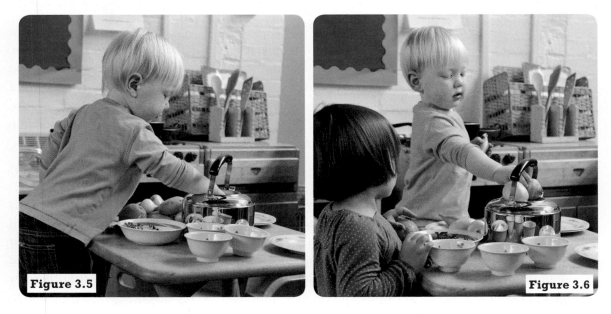

**Figure 3.5**

**Figure 3.6**

William takes the vegetables and fruit (small potatoes, baby onions, an orange and a lemon) and heaps them onto the table. He is deeply engrossed as he then places them in the kettle (see Figure 3.5).

Samira, age 2 years 8 months, joins him. He continues to fill the kettle until it is too full to put the lid on (see Figure 3.6).

Then Samira starts to unpack the kettle into the bowls. She is talking to him and he replies with much conversational intonation, but as yet few recognisable words. He then puts the cup to the spout of the kettle as if to fill it up.

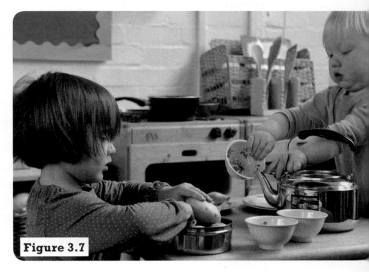

**Figure 3.7**

### What have we found out?

The rich provision in this home corner, with recently added new resources (real vegetables and fruit) motivates William to become deeply involved in his explorations. As he is just 19 months old there are not yet that many recognisable words in his speech, but he replies to Samira with enthusiasm. Towards the end of the observation we see how his exploration is turning into pretend play, as he pretends to fill up the cup.

### Samira, age 2 years 8 months

Samira, who is in the under-3s room in a Children's Centre, has been taken by her key person to explore the larger and more challenging garden for the older children. She sees some of the children she knows as they had been in the under-3s room with her until a few months earlier.

She explores the soft play blocks and begins to build a house, making a rectangular enclosure. She invites two children she knows to her party in the house, showing them the windows and doors and the party food. She leaves the house and finds a buggy, which she climbs into. One of the children she has been playing with pushes her around. Soon they return to the soft blocks, this time attempting to build a bridge. Samira goes off towards the slide. She joins a small group waiting for their turn, and says "1, 2, 3, go" as each child slides down.

### What have we found out?

The garden is quite new to Samira as she is a visitor to the older children's area. She demonstrates confidence to explore quite a wide area in the large garden and get involved in play with a small group of older children she already knows. The nursery's plans for her now include regular visits to the large garden area, thinking about the resourcing of their own home corner and opportunities and encouragement to build. The environment and the support from her key person has helped her to feel sufficiently at ease to become deeply involved in building and to participate with others.

## What the experts say
### Listening and outdoor play

### Observation, assessment and planning: Listening to children

An important aspect of observing and assessing young children is listening to them: their views about themselves and their own learning matter! These need to be incorporated into planning for them, but being able to reflect on their own learning and express what they think and feel to others is difficult for young children. Many might think it is impossible for babies and toddlers who are only at the very beginning of learning to communicate. However, in recent years a great deal of work has been done on how we might effectively gather children's views.

In England an influential project was the Coram Family Listening to Young Children project, which grew out of work by Alison Clark and Peter Moss, first reported in 2001. The project examined ways of helping even the very youngest to communicate their preferences, for example, by helping children to use child-friendly digital cameras to record what is important to them about their setting. A set of training materials were developed as a result of this project and many settings used this to develop the children's ability to reflect on their own learning. There are some useful case studies of settings involving children in the assessment process in Hutchin (2007, 2012), as well as later in this book (see Chapter 16).

## The learning environment: Outdoors

The increasing emphasis on young children learning outdoors has been overwhelmingly endorsed by the EYFS and by professionals working with children and families, especially early years practitioners. As a result there are now many exciting projects involving practitioners and parents working together, not just to enhance the environment, but to ensure better use of it to support children's learning.

A notable advocate for outdoor play is Jan White, who has written and edited several books about the importance of outdoor play, as well as working with Siren Films to make three excellent DVD packs demonstrating the learning of babies, toddlers and 2-year-olds in stimulating outdoor provision. As she says:

*"play outdoors offers children:*

- *access to space with opportunities to be their natural, exuberant, physical and noisy selves*
- *fresh air and direct experience of how the elements and weather feel*
- *contact with natural and living things...*
- *freedom to be inquisitive, exploratory, adventurous, innovative and messy..."*

(White, 2009)

## Effective practice:
## What do we need to do?

### Observation, assessment and planning

#### Observing

Use a mix of methods for observing, depending on what you are doing at the time:

- Quick, short notes as you are working with children are very useful; it is also useful to note things you see that you were not involved in but that seem to be significant.
- Narrative observations are invaluable. This means standing back for three to four minutes to watch when the child is engrossed in a child-initiated activity. Many settings find one narrative observation every few weeks provides enough information, together with the other ongoing notes, to plan effectively. You will find more information about all these types of observations in Chapter 16. Observations should always be positive, showing achievements and what the child is exploring and trying out, with plans for what comes next.

### Recording and reviewing

- Ensure you have a daily review meeting with other staff at the end of each day or session, to recap on the day and ensure planning is right for the next day. If staff are working shifts, make sure there is a quick handover chat to inform another member of staff who is there until the end of the day about what your key children have been doing, so this can be passed on to parents.
- Review records of your key children regularly so you can pull together all you know about each child's learning and development. See Chapter 10 for more information.

### Sharing

- Store your records accessibly so children and parents can share them. Plastic document wallets for each sheet help to keep them clean and waterproof. There should be nothing confidential in these records.
- Ensure parents know they can look at their child's record with them. Make regular appointments with parents to discuss the child's development in more depth, so that you can both share what you know and plan the possibilities and opportunities to provide next.

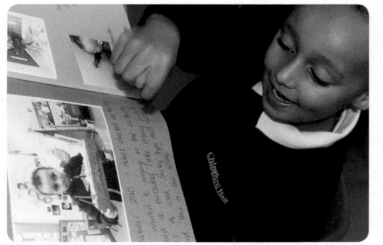

**Figure 3.8** Brandon is looking at his own super book (his learning diary), which is displayed accessibly in the room

### Planning

- Make sure your planning is responsive to what has been happening, the child's particular interests or indeed lack of interest. A lack of interest from the children means something needs to be changed, such as greater adult involvement or a better enabling environment.
- Do not forget to plan the books and stories you will be using – prepare for your story and song time.

## The learning environment: Continuous provision

Much of what is provided to create a rich and stimulating learning environment is through what many people call 'continuous provision'. This is the planning that enables successful child-initiated learning to take place. It requires careful planning to ensure that it is appropriate and tailored to the children's learning and development needs.

# Keeping the environment rich and stimulating for under-3s

*For babies*:

- Ensure there are plenty of natural materials for them to experience. So many toys these days are plastic, but babies need a variety of textures to feel. They learn through using *all* their senses. Remember they use their mouths to touch, feel and taste, so resources need to be washed regularly, and watch out for items that could be swallowed, or worse, stuck in the throat.
- Outside, babies need different sensory experiences: surfaces to feel and crawl on, as well as scented plants to smell, the wind to feel, the trees to see.

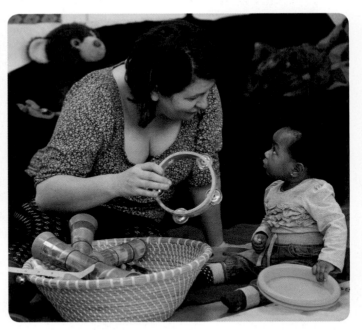

**Figure 3.9** A basket full of safe percussion toys with the key person supporting

*For toddlers*:

- Toddlers generally want to explore everything and make use of all available space, both indoors and outdoors. Much of the resources and environment for older children can be provided for toddlers, taking account of safety since a lot of exploration is still done by putting objects in their mouths. This is the age where symbolic play and role play really start, so a well-set-up home corner area, with dressing up, plenty of bags as well as small world toys, are needed.

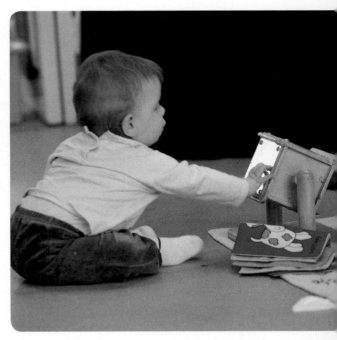

**Figure 3.10** Mirrors are a special educational attraction for babies

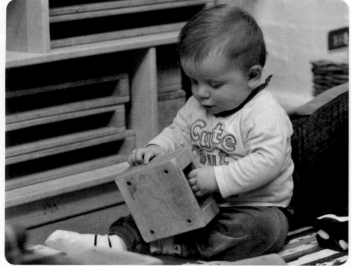

**Figure 3.11** Babies and toddlers are fascinated by the properties of materials

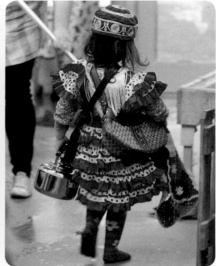

**Figure 3.12** Bags and dressing up are a particular interest for some children, especially the "transporters"

## Helpful tip

Every practitioner needs to take responsibility for keeping the environment clean, safe and looking attractive and inviting. Here are some suggestions to help achieve this:

➤ It is helpful to use photographs and words when labelling boxes.

➤ Encourage children to help tidy up as they go along.

➤ Where children are finding it difficult to get used to certain routines, such as keeping the bathroom tidy or being careful with each other on the climbing frame or sharing wheel toys, devise a set of rules *with* the children so that they have been involved in the decision making.

➤ Involve children in caring for and, where possible, mending resources, for example, if a book has been torn.

## Activity

Take photographs of an area of your setting that is particularly troublesome to keep tidy, showing the sequence of a tidying-up routine, such as how to hang up coats or store wellington boots. Laminate and display the photographs in the appropriate spot so that children can remind each other of what they need to do.

## Indoor environment for 3 to 5-year-olds

The learning environment is also an important teacher, and depends upon careful presentation and thoughtful planning.

*"When the environment is right, there is a contagious sparkle in the air, the children are deeply engaged in their learning and practitioners' confidence soars as they are free to support each child constructively on their learning journey."*

(Jaeckle, 2008)

### Indoor resources

Important indoor resources for firing children's imagination whilst also educating them include:

- book areas that are attractive and well cared for to grab the children's interest
- a range of tools to use and different materials for connecting, such as cardboard, paper, scissors, sticky tape and glue
- interesting recycled resources to make things with, such as cardboard packaging, boxes, string and cellophane.

Other excellent resources are shown in the photos below and on the following page:

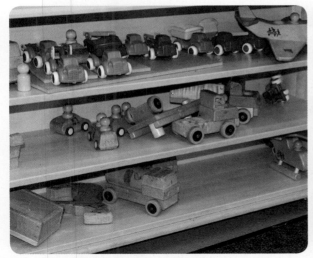

**Figure 3.13 Small world:** an attractive presentation of resources, which can easily be returned to their place

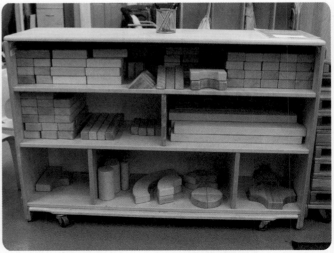

**Figure 3.14 Wooden block area:** If the attribute blocks are not carefully displayed then children cannot see their mathematical qualities or potential for building

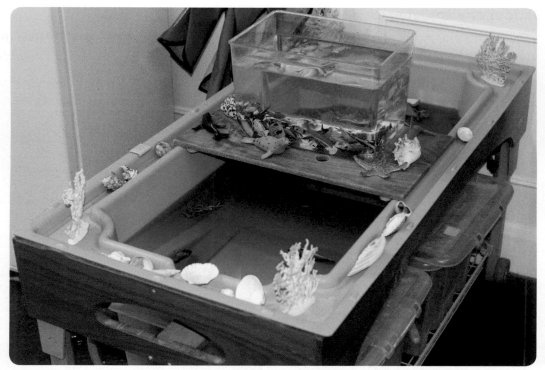

**Figure 3.15 Water and sand**: inviting, imaginative and attractive provision will spark imagination as well as support thinking and experimenting

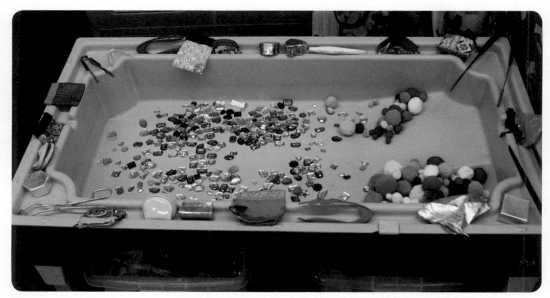

**Figure 3.16 Firing the imagination**: jewels, tweezers and purses in a dry water tray

## Outdoors: inspiration and challenge

There are many outdoor opportunities for children, which will inspire and challenge them. Waterproof gear (raincoats and Wellington boots), ensures children can be outside in all weathers.

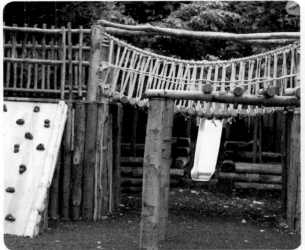

**Figure 3.17** Challenging fixed equipment provides opportunities to climb, prance, balance and swing

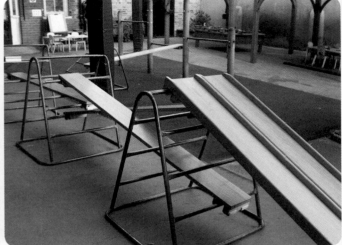

**Figure 3.18** Challenging climbing equipment that can be taken apart and used in other ways

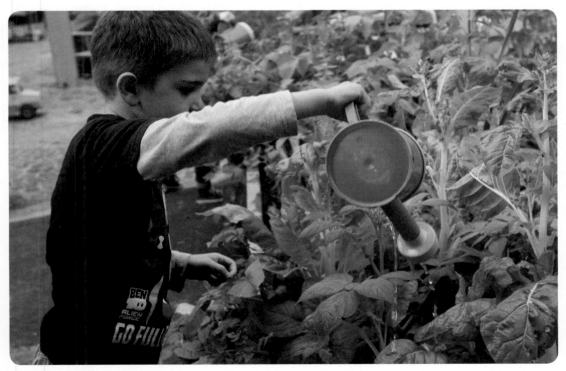

**Figure 3.19** Growing vegetables provides an important learning opportunity

## Case study: St Anne's Nursery School and Children's Centre

Before the children and parents arrive in the mornings, St Anne's Nursery School and Children's Centre is a hive of activity, as the team thoughtfully prepares the environment to enrich learning and development across the spectrum of EYFS. The atmosphere of busy, focused and friendly teamwork is palpable. The outdoor area is as meticulously planned and prepared as the indoor area. The continuous provision, as well as being tailored to the interests of the children, also introduces new experiences to them. When children arrive they immediately immerse themselves in play, investigate and explore new ideas, persist in trying out new skills, pose their own challenges, as well as get involved in the adult-framed experiences presented by the practitioners. This is a truly enabling environment.

## Case study: Woodlands Park Children's Centre and learning outdoors

Walking into the large, inspiring and deliberately challenging garden at Woodlands Park, the thought and planning that has gone into it is obvious. It has taken a few years to build up, but this vibrant garden is full of life, with its shady wooded area, one or two small trees to climb, wooden monkey bars and a demanding climbing wall, wooden swing bridge and quiet secluded areas that fire children's imagination. Next to it is an asphalt area, a water feature where water cascades through a series of pools, with the tap accessible to the children, and a sand pit. The staff have recently added a vegetable garden using old railway sleepers, where children plant, care for and eat their own vegetables. (For information on how the Centre carries out its risk assessments to ensure the garden is safe, see the case study in Chapter 1.)

Children can access the garden for most of the day, every day, in all weathers, free-flowing between indoors and outdoors. The staff team are well aware of the vast opportunities for learning provided by the outdoor area and, most importantly, the role of the adult within it. Their outdoor play policy states:

*"Outdoor play works well when it is supported and enjoyed by all staff. The effective adult:*
- *is mobile and vigilant*
- *encourages play*
- *challenges children to try out ideas*
- *values creative ideas*
- *stresses independence*
- *is optimistic about outcomes*
- *shows real interest*
- *actively listens*
- *accepts children's decisions*
- *follows children's interests*
- *uses open questions."*

(Outdoor play policy statement, Woodlands Park Children's Centre)

The garden is checked over every morning before the children arrive and resources set out as necessary. Assigning specific roles to staff outside is key to ensuring the garden provides a rich learning environment for every child, including those with additional needs. Three members of staff are involved at all times outside, one positioned to support play at either end, and a "floater" who is "to be flexible, moving between areas supervising and interacting with the children".

## Chapter summary

This chapter will have helped you:
➤ understand the EYFS principle and commitments for Enabling Environments
➤ think about how observation is important not only in assessing children's learning, but for planning too
➤ reflect on the learning environment in your own setting and the role the environment plays in supporting children's learning and development.

## Further reading and references

Clark, A., and Moss, P. (2001) *Listening to Young Children: The Mosiac Approach*, National Children's Bureau and Joseph Rowntree Foundation

Hutchin, V. (2007) *Supporting Every Child's Learning in the EYFS*, Hodder Education, London

Hutchin, V. (2012) *Assessing and Supporting Young Children's Learning in the EYFS*, Hodder Education, London

Jaeckle, S. (2008) 'The EYFS Principles: A Breakdown', *Early Years Update*, Optimus Education, London (www.teachingexpertise.com/articles/eyfs-principles-breakdown-4117)

Lancaster, Y.P. and Kirby, P. (2010) Coram Family Listening to Young Children pack, Open University Press

White, J. (2009) *Playing and Learning Outdoors: Making Provision for High Quality Experiences in the Outdoor Environment*, Nursery World/Routledge Essential Guides: Guides for Early Years Practitioners, Routledge, London

### Useful websites

Common Assessment Framework: www.cwdcouncil.org.uk/caf

Learning through Landscapes: www.ltl.org.uk

Siren Films: www.sirenfilms.co.uk

# Chapter 4

# Learning and Development

## In this chapter we will be looking at:

➤ the principle of Learning and Development, which covers *how* children learn as well as *what* we want them to learn, with an emphasis on the final commitment, Areas of learning and development

➤ the differences between the prime and the specific areas of learning

➤ observations of children learning and developing through play, emphasising what as well as how they are learning

➤ some key experts on how children learn

➤ ensuring our practice is effective in supporting learning.

## Introduction

This chapter begins by looking at the first three commitments of Learning and Development, which consider *how* children learn. In the EYFS 2012 these are called the "characteristics of effective learning", and they form the topics covered in Section 2. We then move on to look at the "areas of learning and development" – *what* we want children to learn. There are seven areas of learning altogether and in this chapter we focus on the differences between the prime and specific areas. Young children's learning is fascinating – how do they manage to learn so much so quickly? To most of us, it seems quite amazing. Let's start by listening to the thoughts of two children who are just 4 years old.

On one of the first cold, wintry days of the year, Vinnie says about the effect of hot weather: "It makes you even tired if the sun is out and it's hot. It makes your head all sweaty." Annie, in another nursery, while watching some chicks hatch, asks: "They look tired. Is there only one chick in the egg? Is that why they're tired because they had to come out all on their own?"

These examples are of young children making sense of the world around them. These are the children's own interpretations and questions: they are not repeating what others say and no one else has said it in this way. How do they come up with these thoughts and ideas, and what are they learning?

## The EYFS principle, Learning and Development, tells us:

*"Children develop and learn in different ways and at different rates. The framework covers the education and care of all children in early years provision, including children with special educational needs and disabilities."*

(EYFS Statutory Framework, 2012)

## What is this theme about?

The theme of Learning and Development looks at *how* children learn and develop (the characteristics of effective learning) as well as *what* we want them to learn (the areas of learning and development). The principle points out that every child is unique and reminds us that the framework for the EYFS is about *all* children and all types of provision. It is inclusive.

Every aspect of learning is interconnected. We often say that children's learning is holistic – it is not compartmentalised into areas of learning but takes place as a whole, covering many aspects at the same time. We may differentiate learning into different areas, but this is to help us ensure that we are providing the breadth of learning opportunities every child needs.

The supporting commitments within Learning and Development fall into two categories. The first three commitments relate to *how* children learn and are given fuller coverage in Section 2 of this book. The final supporting commitment is about *what* children learn.

The four commitments are:
- Playing and exploring
- Active learning
- Creating and thinking critically
- Areas of learning and development.

The Tickell Review in 2011 called the first three commitments the "characteristics of learning". The EYFS Statutory Framework 2012 asks all reception teachers to provide the Year 1 teachers with information addressing the characteristics of learning for each child, but they are very important to all practitioners as they are about how children learn. Because these are so important we have devoted Section 2 of the book entirely to them, but we also look briefly at them here.

## How children learn: Playing and exploring

*"Children's play reflects their wide ranging and varied interests and preoccupations. In their play children learn and develop at their highest level. Play with peers is important for children's development."*

(EYFS card 4.1)

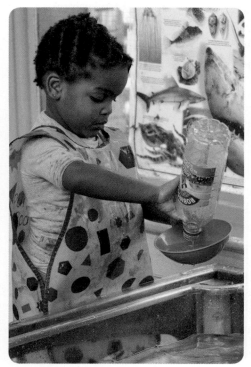

**Figure 4.1** This 2-year-old has spent 20 minutes exploring the flow of water, concentrating deeply

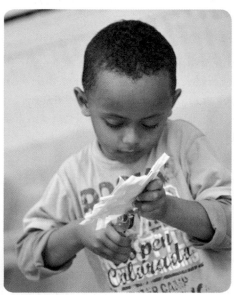

**Figure 4.2** This boy is deeply involved in thinking through what he is creating

Play is fun, but it is not *just* fun. It has a very serious purpose as a main vehicle for children's learning. It enables children to be in charge and in control of what goes on in their play. They use their imagination, express their own ideas and follow their own lines of enquiry, experiment, practise skills and apply what they know. Through play they can relive past experiences and try out things they have seen others do. As Tina Bruce puts it in one of her books on play:

*"Children at play are able to stay flexible, respond to events and changing situations, be sensitive to people, to adapt and think on their feet and keep altering what they do in a fast-moving scene."*

(Bruce, 2001)

Playing and exploring is the topic of Chapter 6 in Section 2 of this book, where you will find a full explanation and many examples of effective practice.

## How children learn: Active learning

*"Children learn best through physical and mental challenges. Active learning involves other people, objects, ideas and events that engage and involve children for sustained periods."*

(EYFS card 4.2)

All learning is active: the children are mentally engaged and fully alert, even if they appear to be quiet and contemplative – we cannot always see the active learning; it is a mental process. As EYFS EP 2008 states:

*"As they come across objects, situations, people and ideas, they adjust and structure their knowledge by trying to make sense of their experiences."*

Active learning is the topic of Chapter 7 in Section 2.

## How children learn: Creating and thinking critically

*"When children have opportunities to play with ideas in different situations and with a variety of resources, they discover connections and come to new and better understandings and ways of doing things. Adult support in this process enhances their ability to think critically and ask questions."*

(EYFS card 4.3)

Children *create* connections for themselves through play, exploring the world around them and interacting with others, and as a result they develop new concepts and refine their ideas. The role of adults in these explorations is vital, providing a rich environment for learning with plenty of opportunities to encourage curiosity, showing a genuine interest and getting involved in exploring alongside the child.

Creating and thinking critically is the topic of Chapter 8 in Section 2.

## What we want children to learn:
## Areas of learning and development

To help us look at the seven areas of learning and how they are organised, here is an example of a carefully set up adult-led activity – a storytelling session – which shows us *how* children's learning works together with *what* children learn. The example describes a story session that was videoed. The video is a very powerful sequence of young children deeply engaged in thinking, showing them expressing their thoughts and ideas and sharing their solutions to problems.

### Case study: A story

Seven children aged between 3 and 4 years have been invited to join a story session about a special doll called a Persona Doll. This particular doll is new to the children and is in a wheelchair. The doll is wheeled into the room in her chair by the practitioner and the children sit down. The practitioner begins by introducing the children to Polly the doll, telling them about her family and that she is 4 years old. This makes a personal and immediate link for the children, as they each in turn tell the doll how old they are. One child asks why she is in a wheelchair and the practitioner explains that Polly cannot walk and that she lives in a bungalow. The camera pans the children's faces. They are wide-eyed and listening intently, concentrating. Their thinking is visible. They begin to ask questions:

"What's a bungalow?" asks one child, and a discussion ensues on what a bungalow is and why Polly needs to live in one. The children make connections, talking about where they live – some in houses, some in flats. This is a new word and a new concept to them all.

Another child asks, "Why can't she walk?" The practitioner's answer is that Polly was born like this, and they discuss the other things she cannot do, such as run, jump and hop. Again the children make connections with what they can do. The practitioner tells them about the races she has in her wheelchair with her brother running beside her. The image of Polly that the practitioner creates is entirely positive, as a competent and able child who has fun like they do. This leads to further discussion and the children seem delighted with this positive game the doll and her brother play.

The practitioner moves the story on to how difficult it is for Polly to go to the local shopping mall because there are steps. The children are invited to find solutions to the problem – what should Polly do? One child mentions the shopping mall he knows that has an escalator. Another problem is posed: how will Polly manage on an escalator? The children suggest the solutions, and one boy who has not spoken before has a lot of ideas to offer, extending the discussion further.

(This example is taken from the *Persona Dolls in Action* video, reproduced with kind permission from Persona Doll Training)

## How they are learning

The short story described in the case study above was devised by the practitioner, using a doll as the main character, and its aim is for children to be able to empathise with others and begin to understand what is meant by inclusion. The children are totally engaged and the practitioner has provided an impressive amount of support to the children's thinking, understanding and problem solving, as she lets the story flow with the responses of these young children. Different children in the group ask different sorts of questions and this shows their unique concerns and interests in the story. They do not all speak; some are quietly listening, but you can still see them thinking. Most of all, the young children were using their imaginations effectively, making connections between Polly's life and their own lives, and also using their critical thinking skills.

Although play is a key vehicle for children's learning it is not the only way that children learn: appropriate adult-led activities are really important too. The case study session is not play. You can see from the description of the video how the children are engaged in active learning and the "mental challenge" referred to in that commitment, as well as how they are using their creativity and critical thinking skills.

## What they are learning

As well as showing how the children are learning, this one story and discussion covered several areas of learning for the children. These children were learning in a natural way as the story and conversation flowed between all the participants. It is only when we look back on it that we can see how many areas and aspects of areas of learning were covered. However, for the children the learning is holistic; it is not divided into areas of learning.

### *Personal, social and emotional development:*

- Developing confidence to talk to others.
- Learning about other people's feelings and developing empathy for others.
- Learning about relationships and making connections between their own lives and other people's.
- Working as part of a group to solve problems.

### *Communication and language:*

- Learning to listen to what the practitioner and the other children are saying.
- Learning new vocabulary, such as wheelchair, bungalow and escalator.
- Learning to express their thoughts and ideas and to talk in a group.

### *Understanding the world:*

- Learning about differences and similarities between people.
- Learning about people and places, different terrains and the problems they may pose for some people.
- Learning about the differences between people through the story presented to them by the practitioner about the doll.
- Learning about technology, its usefulness and limitations, for example, the wheelchair.

## The EYFS areas of learning

In 2011 changes were proposed to look at the areas of learning in a new way, which really helps take our thinking further about how, as well as what, children learn. Rather than stating that all areas of learning are of equal importance, it acknowledged that there are differences in nature between some of the areas of learning. It has designated some as *prime areas of learning* and others as *specific areas of learning*. Why has this been done?

In 2009 a useful document was produced by the government that reviewed the latest research on children's learning and development. This was the 'Early Years Learning and Development: Literature Review' (Evangelou *et al.*, 2009). As well as emphasising that children's learning is *holistic*, the review highlighted the "centrality" of personal, social and emotional development, communication and language and physical development, and how these are fundamental to children's development. As the Tickell Review put it: "Children are primed to encounter their environment through relating to and communicating with others and engaging physically in their experiences" (Tickell, 2011). These three areas of learning are now called the prime areas of learning.

## The prime areas of learning

The three prime areas of learning are:
1 Personal, social and emotional development
2 Communication and language
3 Physical development.

The prime areas of learning and development relate very closely to child development and are universal to every child across the world, regardless of their social or cultural context. As the Tickell Review stated: "These (areas of learning) play a crucial role… in laying the cornerstones for healthy development. Without secure development in these particular areas during this critical period, children will struggle to progress" (Tickell, 2011).

## Child development

Children want to communicate as well as to explore the world physically. Research shows that these prime areas relate to the developing brain from the earliest stages – pre-birth onwards. They are time-sensitive: "if not securely in place by the age of five, they will be more difficult to acquire and their absence may hold the child back in other areas of learning" (Tickell, 2011).

These areas of development are interdependent and interconnected, as children use their physical, social and communicative abilities at the same time. Each of the prime areas of learning is the focus of a chapter – see Chapters 9, 10 and 11. The prime areas of learning also interconnect with the four other specific areas of learning.

## The specific areas of learning

Dependent on the prime areas of learning are the other four areas of learning:

1 Literacy
2 Mathematics (previously called Problem-solving, reasoning and numeracy)
3 Understanding the world (previously called Knowledge and understanding of the world)
4 Expressive arts and design (previously called Creative development).

These areas of learning are different in nature to the prime areas. They relate more to bodies of knowledge than the prime areas and are something that in modern life we all *wish* children to be learning – they do not come naturally. As the Tickell Review points out: "These specific areas of learning are influenced by the times we live in and our beliefs about what it is important for children to learn" (Tickell, 2011).

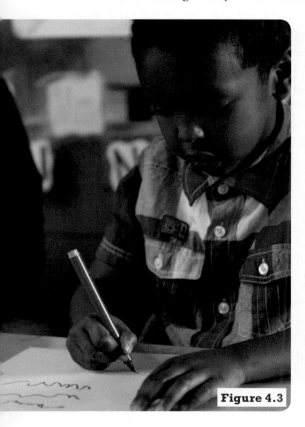

**Figure 4.3**

There are two technical terms used in the Tickell Review that are quoted from research and help to explain the differences between the prime and the specific: "experience expectant" and "experience dependent". The prime areas are experience expectant: "the brain *expects* certain kinds of input to which it will adapt itself". However, in the specific areas of learning, learning does not occur by itself, but is experience dependent, that is, dependent on children deliberately being given certain experiences to help them learn, such as access to books and being regularly and frequently read to. Chapters 12–15 in Section 4 look at these specific areas of learning.

It is important to remember, however, that it is not a question of first the prime areas of learning and then the specific; the development of the specific areas begins as we introduce babies and toddlers to a wide range of experiences, such as the world of books and objects to explore. Let us now see how the areas of learning are interconnected in practice through some observations of individual children learning. You will see the children learning in both the prime and the specific areas of learning.

## Looking at children:
## What do we see?

### Freddie, age 3 years

Freddie was on his own with a box of farm animals and small world people. He lined up the animals, making animal noises. Another child came along and tried to take the donkey from him: "No, it's my donkey". He continued lining up the animals next to the train track. A different child starts to play and this time Freddie is happy to share the animals with her. He looked through the other drawers and became very excited when he found a kangaroo. He placed it on the train track bridge and then began to read books to it that he found nearby. He showed the pictures to the animals and then started to sing to them, "Dancing, dancing kangaroo, dancing where are you?" He began to fix the train together, putting people onto the train, saying, "Mummy on train, mummy got train, mummy go to work now, on the train, mummy gone now." The play continues for some time and Freddie remains absorbed in it on his own.

### What have we found out?

#### How he is learning

Freddie, at 3 years, is beginning to get more deeply involved in imaginative play with objects – in this case animals and trains. He is also busy exploring the resources, looking into the boxes to see what he can find. He is integrating this with his love of books and mimicking reading to the animals. His learning is holistic as it flows from one thing to the next.

#### What he is learning

- *Personal, social and emotional development:* Freddie is able to be assertive when a child tries to take something from him, but also inclusive of another child. He rehearses the adult role in his play as he reads to the animals, and also in his play on the train.
- *Communication and language:* He uses short phrases to communicate at the appropriate level for his age and one phrase is five words long. He uses language to express his imaginary conversation as well as to pretend to read stories. He remembers the words of a rhyme.
- *Literacy:* Freddie shows his developing literacy skills as well as interest in books. This includes using a reading behaviour: showing his audience the pictures in the book. He sings a song that he remembers.

- *Understanding the world:* He is demonstrating his knowledge of animals and their names, knowing donkey and kangaroo. He is also familiar with trains as something that transports Mummies to work.
- *Expressive arts and design*: Freddie is using his imagination to act out a story he is creating in his head. This is sometimes called symbolic play: using one thing to stand for another – in this case, the animals stand in for real animals or people who have Mummies.

### Rosie age 3 years 4 months and Tamarah in role play

Rosie is playing with Tamarah, an older child who she often chooses to play with. They are in the office corner outside, which is set up with computer keyboards, a variety of telephones, clipboards, notepads and an appointments book. Rosie is on the phone, acting out a telephone conversation in a very convincing way. Another child comes up, talking at the girls at a high volume. Still in role, Rosie speaks into the telephone and says to her pretend recipient: "Someone is shouting at me. No? No, it not your Mum."

Tamarah: "That's not my mum?"
Rosie to Tamarah: "I don't know your Mum's number. You do it." She hands the phone to Tamara and begins to type on the keyboard. Tamarah passes the phone back.
Tamarah: "Is that not your Mum? Is it your friend then?"
Rosie types on the keyboard, then picks up the mobile phone: "It's my mum. No, I think it is Sean. Hello! Hello, Sean, are you still at the school?"
Tamarah: "That's just a pretend phone. I have a real computer."
Rosie: "I have too."
Tamarah: "No you haven't."
Rosie: "Let's swap in a minute."

Tamarah begins to type vigorously, using one finger per key, and as she does so she speaks out loud what she is typing, clearly articulating the words in time with her typing. Rosie goes back to using the mobile: "I'm going to the hairdresser." As she talks into the mobile she puts her hand over her other ear, looking very much like an adult in a noisy place trying to hear on the phone.

### What have we found out?

#### How they are learning

These two children are both demonstrating the power of role play in learning and development. To the observer the play seems very serious indeed – and very real to the children. They are both deeply involved in the play and, through it, exploring what it might be like to be an adult in an office. However, although all the mannerisms are of adult behaviour – Rosie's telephone manner and Tamarah's typing – much of the talk is about what they know, about mums and a brother at school.

#### What they are learning

- *Personal, social and emotional development:* The children relate successfully to each other, accommodating each other's points of view to keep the play going.
- *Communication and language:* They listen, speak and understand each other, and Rosie uses language in role on the telephone.

- *Expressive arts and design:* The children are using their imaginations highly effectively to get into role and imagine they are in an office, but they are also able to flip in and out of role as they talk about the resources. They also show their awareness of technology, as they are actually using real telephones (disconnected!) and real computer keyboards.

### Activity

Observe one child, a pair of children or a group playing for three to four minutes, either inside or outside. How many areas of learning and aspects within these did you notice as you analysed the observation?

## What the experts say
## Social learning and babies' brains

Studying child development as we know it first began in the late 18th to early 19th century, through studies such as those by Charles Darwin, and later, in the 20th century, by others such as Jean Piaget and Lev Vygotsky. This tradition of child studies continues to be important in developing our knowledge, now often with the use of video.

### Learning is social

The famous Russian child psychologist, Lev Vygotsky, writing in the 1930s, is often quoted as his work has been so influential to our modern-day early childhood education. He died very young, but ever since his theories were translated into English in the 1960s they have made a huge difference to our understanding of children's learning. Much of his research was from observing children in everyday situations. He understood the importance of play in children's learning: in play children operate at their highest level, "… beyond his average age, above his daily behaviour; in play it is as though he were a head taller than himself" (Vygotsky, 1978). The EYFS commitment for Playing and exploring relates directly to Vygotsky's work.

Vygotsky believed that learning takes place in a social context and is actively constructed by the child: children do not learn by being told

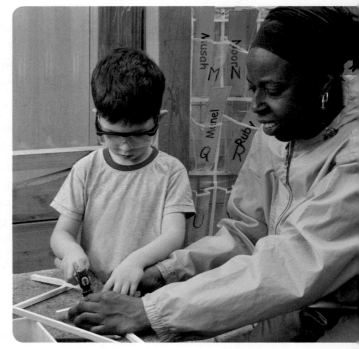

**Figure 4.4** What a child can do with help today, he can do alone tomorrow

something, they have to make it their own. His most well-known theory is about the role that others can play in helping a child to learn. To make a difference the support needs to be in the right way at the right time for the individual child. As Dame Clare Tickell put it in the EYFS Review 2011, "this support is the difference between what a child can do on their own and what they can do when guided by someone else ..." (Tickell, 2011)

What a child can do on his or her own is seen as the child's actual development. But, so long as the help is in tune with the child's own individual development, what a child can do with help now, he or she will be able to do alone in the future. The gap between the actual development and what a child can do with help, Vygotsky calls the zone of proximal development (sometimes called potential development). Planning for play and planning for how practitioners will get involved in supporting the learning is dependent on knowing the children well and knowing the right amount of support to give.

## Babies are brilliant thinkers

Since around 1980 we have found out a great deal from research on brain development, including the vital role that caring adults, especially the mother, play in shaping the baby's brain. From the moment of birth the baby develops and learns as a result of the nurturing she or he receives from close, loving relationships, and the warmth, comfort and safety provided.

Alison Gopnik and her colleagues Andrew Meltzoff and Patricia Kuhl are professors of psychology in the USA. They are internationally recognised for their work on children's learning and development, particularly about how babies think. Their book, *How Babies Think* (2001) is an accessible, light-hearted but serious book about the latest research in how babies develop, aimed primarily at parents, but just as useful for professionals and students working with young children. In the book the authors show us how the most recent research about babies' developing brains is transforming our ideas about them: "... the new research shows us that babies and young children learn more about the world than we could ever have imagined. They think, draw conclusions, make predictions, look for explanations and even do experiments" (Gopnik *et al.* 2001).

They summarise much of the research about how young babies learn so quickly about the world around them, as well as the importance of relationships and language. Babies do all of this through playing and exploring, using all their senses and movement, but also as a result of the close relationships with their main carers. Gopnik shows us how a sequence becomes established very quickly, whereby babies learn from what their carers do, and carers then learn from the baby's response how to respond appropriately. As this process continues, so does the development of the child.

## Supporting how children learn

### Playing and exploring

- Make sure you provide an environment that supports children's play and exploration, taps into their interests and builds on these to ensure there are exciting new opportunities for further learning.

### Active learning

- Know the children well so that you can provide the kind of challenges that will motivate them. Active learning is about mental as well as physical challenges.

### Creating and thinking critically

- Have informal discussions regularly with children. If they ask you "why" questions, figure out the answers *with* the children, supporting them to create their own investigations and problems to solve. Children, like adults, can learn as much, if not more, from their mistakes than they do from getting things right. This will encourage them to ask more questions and to investigate.

### Areas of learning and development

- Remember that play is the main vehicle for children's learning. Plan interesting and inviting continuous provision for play and child-initiated learning inside and outside, so that all areas of learning are covered. This means planning for both the prime and specific areas of learning, regardless of the EYFS age range of the children you are catering for.
- Plan the practitioner role in your daily and weekly plans: in other words, which practitioner does what, where and when. Make sure there are practitioners who will be supporting play and children's self-chosen activities inside and outside, as well as adult-led activities.
- Be flexible and make sure every planned adult-led activity is playful and fun.
- Remember children's learning is not compartmentalised into different areas of learning. They are learning in many areas and aspects of learning at the same time. In a cooking activity, for example, they may learn about the science of cooking (how the dry ingredients change as they mix with liquids or eggs, and change again once cooked) and about number as they count spoonfuls of ingredients, but the children may also be learning:
  - about taking turns
  - to listen to instructions
  - new vocabulary
  - to develop their own descriptive words to describe consistency
  - physical skills, such as stirring.

Reflect on how the areas of learning are covered in your setting. Are there areas of learning that have particular strengths? Are there areas of learning that you think need further development?

## Case study: Developing planning at Fiveways Play Centre: A new way of working

Fiveways Play Centre is a parent-run, voluntary-sector, preschool playgroup, which takes children from 2 years 6 months until they go into reception class. It has recently moved into a new, open-plan building with easy access to outdoor provision. The managers said:

*"The open plan nature of the new building means that we needed more regular planning meetings than before to make sure it all works well. The children have access to every space and they free-flow between indoors and outdoors. We were in two separate rooms before, with two small teams, so it was quite different. Now we have four key groups for the children and the staff responsible for each group meet once a week to plan. They choose the time that suits them best: some meet at the end of the day, others at lunchtime."*

Observations are written on sticky notes as the staff work with the children, and these are then compiled into the children's learning journals, with photographs and the children's work.

This term they are trialling a new short-term planning approach. If the staff find something is not working well, they are happy to review it and address the issues. The staff team is highly experienced and knows the EYFS well, and is confident that they are providing for all areas of learning. For long-term planning the setting uses the format devised by their local authority, based around planning to meet the themes and commitments of the EYFS. This works well. The Room Leader told me:

*"The short-term planning we do now is much more targeted at the specific learning needs and interests of the children than it used to be."*

The aim is to involve parents and the children as much as possible in the planning. The children's ideas for planning are gathered at a key group circle time every few weeks. Their ideas are written onto large paper for all to see and these then form the basis for the play provision and child-initiated activities.

At the previous parents' evening, parents were asked about what they wanted their children to be learning. When all the parents' ideas were collated, the Room Leader realised that every area of learning was covered very well!

*"This will form the basis of our adult-led activities this term. We used to do topic planning, but I think this will work much better as we are addressing our children's real needs and interests and working more closely with the parents too."*

## Chapter summary

This chapter will have helped you:

➤ understand why the areas of learning are seen as prime or specific and the differences between them

➤ understand the importance of how children learn to ensure your practice is effective

➤ recognise that children's learning is holistic and integrated – they do not learn in compartmentalised subjects

➤ find out about some important research about learning.

## Further reading and references

Bruce, T. (2011) *Learning through Play: For babies, toddlers and young children*, Hodder Education, London

Evangelou, M., Sylva, K., Kyriacou, M., Wild, M. and Glenny, G. (2009) 'Early Years Learning and Development: Literature Review', DCSF Research Report RR176. Available to download from: www.education.gov.uk/publications/RSG/publicationDetail/Page1/DCSF-RR176

Gopnik, A., Meltzoff, A. and Kuhl, K.P. (2001) *How Babies Think*, Orion Publishing Group, London

Tickell, C. (2011) *The Early Years: Foundations for Life, Health And Learning. An Independent Report on the Early Years Foundation Stage to Her Majesty's Government*, Annex 9, p.92. Available to download from: www.education.gov.uk

Vygotsky, L. (1978) *Mind in Society*, Harvard University Press, Harvard

### Useful websites

Persona Doll Training: www.persona-doll-training.org

## Chapter 5

# Developing strong partnerships with parents and carers

## In this chapter we will be looking at:

➤ the EYFS commitment Parents as Partners, and why there is a new emphasis on this

➤ observations of children learning and their parents' views about their learning and the settings they attend

➤ what some key experts tell us about the importance partnerships with parents play in supporting children's learning

➤ what we do to ensure our practice is effective in developing partnerships with every child's family.

## Introduction

Developing partnerships with parents has been seen increasingly as an important factor in children's achievements throughout their time in school as well as in the early years. Partnership means doing things together with each party contributing. It means working together with a common purpose and in this case the common purpose is providing the best for the child.

### The EYFS commitment, Parents as Partners, tells us:

"Parents are children's first and most enduring educators. When parents and practitioners work together in early years settings, the results have a positive impact on children's development and learning."

(EYFS card 2.2)

Let us start by looking at Hetti, 16 months, settling in to her nursery setting. Before Hetti started, her key person and another member of staff visited her at home. The home visit is a really useful way for the nursery staff, particularly the key person, to begin to get to know the child and family before the child starts, in a place where the child feels secure – at home. Hetti played happily with her key person while the other practitioner and Hetti's mother discussed what happens at nursery. For the first few days in the setting, Hetti appeared to settle well, so her mum began to leave her with her key person. But then she started to get upset. No one was quite sure what had changed for her: was it because the nursery seemed busy, especially in the morning when other children were arriving and other parents were coming and going? Her mother found it very upsetting to leave her in this way.

The practitioners thought of strategies to help. Gradually Hetti began to feel more at ease, helped by the photos of her with her family at home that were displayed on the wall within reach. Her key person also suggested that her mother might like to bring in something from home that felt, looked and smelt familiar. This seemed to help too. The daily feedback discussions between her key person and her mother were vital: her key person learned the songs that Hetti enjoyed at home, and through plenty of discussions the nursery was able to fine-tune things just right for her. Very soon she was happy and confident and making friends with others.

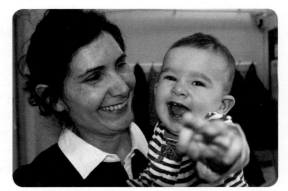

**Figure 5.1** A joyful start to the day

## What is this commitment about?

For young babies, totally dependent on the care they are given, the family, and particularly parents, are the centre of their universe. Even if a baby or child is cared for by others from 8 a.m. to 6 p.m., five days a week, this still amounts to less than one-third of the week, and most children will spend the majority of the rest of their time with their parents. In order to ensure continuity for the child, partnership is vital. What happens at home matters a great deal to children. As it says on the EYFS card 2.2, "Parents and practitioners have a lot to learn from each other."

### Parents as Partners: An area for development

In 2007 an Ofsted report on early years settings noted that although parents were often involved at the beginning of the child's time in the setting, there was little involvement beyond then. The Tickell Review on the EYFS (2011) sees partnership with parents as something we all need to do better.

Even the best settings will usually agree that there is always more they can do to ensure an equal partnership with all parents. Whether you are a practitioner in a setting with many years' experience, a childminder at home or a childcare student, you have undoubtedly chosen to work with children in their early years because you wish to work with young children, not because you chose to work with parents.

What can parents and practitioners learn from each other? To provide the best for the children, we need close links with parents, not only to find out what they do with their children at home so that these can be built on, but also to support parents by using our knowledge of child development and how children learn. The partnership between home and family is vital, with a two-way flow of information, sharing experience and expertise.

## Building trust

Parenthood is a most challenging undertaking:

*"Being a mother or father is to have the most difficult job in the world. As a new parent, you are suddenly responsible for another person, one who is initially totally dependent on you but then begins to assert his or her own personality. ... Bringing a child to an EYFS provision can be the first extended daily contact parents have with childcare professionals. Mothers, fathers and carers may feel that this is a time when they are judged on their parenting skills not just once but on a twice daily basis."*

(National Strategies/DCSF, 2010)

Practitioners often say that parents are not keen to be involved in the setting, that they "don't have time" or are "not interested in what their child has been doing". However, this is most unlikely to be true in reality – it may be fear of being judged or just trying to juggle many priorities. We need to start from the point that every parent has a huge interest and concern about their child, and try to find the best way we can build a partnership with them.

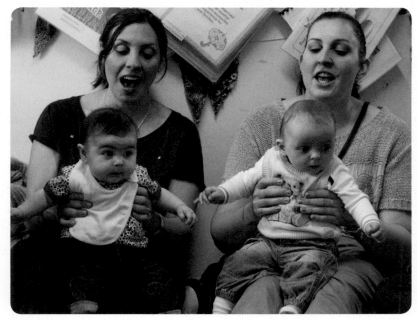

**Figure 5.2** Music and singing is a great way to get parents involved

Valuing every family is easier to say than do – it is all too easy to think that the way we bring up our own children or the way our parents brought us up was the right way to do it. We do this without realising it. There are many acceptable ways of bringing up children and every family is different. When it comes to families that have many differences from our own, we can easily make incorrect assumptions about them. Developing closer relationships with parents is a key way to undo these incorrect assumptions.

## Looking at children:
### What do we see?

In this chapter the observations of children were taken in the home environment. They also include discussions with parents, recording their own views of their child's development and both their own and their child's experiences of being in an early years setting.

## Ives, age 5 years

Ives and his family live in the countryside, very near the sea. From a few months old he has been looked after for some of the time by his grandparents, while both his parents work. As soon as he could walk he was interested in what his grandfather was doing outside, working in the garden or fixing cars, motorbikes and, most of all, boats. A lot of his time is spent right by the sea with his grandparents or his family, and they have supported his interest in boats. By the time he was 4 years, Ives could row a small dinghy himself, closely supervised by his grandfather, and by the age of 5 he could actually row his

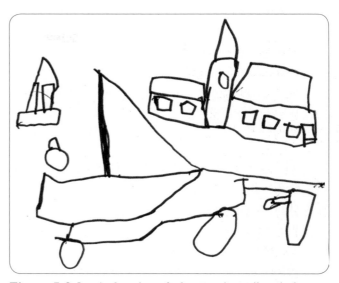

**Figure 5.3** Ives's drawing of a boat on its trailer, tied to a post

grandfather in the boat. He knows a lot about dinghies as well as the sea, tides and wind. Ives's experiences and the skills he has learned are unique to him. He started at a preschool at 2 years 9 months, just one day a week. At 3 years 9 months he changed to a five-day-a-week place in another preschool when his family moved house.

## The parents' perspective: choosing a playgroup

*"For both playgroups we made definite choices – by visiting other playgroups too. I chose the second playgroup because the staff were so welcoming and we could see how the staff were interacting so well with the children. It also had very close links with the local school which he would be moving on to. In our minds were the thoughts: 'Will he be happy here?' 'Do they have the kind of things he would like?' 'What is the outdoor space like and what about construction toys and trikes?' They had all of these things. On our first visit there was a table full of leaves and tree bark and children were hunting for bugs – we knew he would enjoy this.*

*"Before he started they asked us all about him and what he was interested in – I told them what he liked doing and they followed it up. So they did creative activities about boats with him and I can remember when they helped him and some others make binoculars out of toilet roll tubes. He loved that. His key person was very good at taking on his interests – and was very approachable for me as a parent. His grandmother often took him and collected him and she found the same; they would really take him into account when deciding what to do."*

## What have we found out?

His parents were very happy with Ives's playgroup and how keen the practitioners were to work with his interests and build on his skills. Through his close relationships within the family he has developed the confidence to learn, among many other things, how to row a boat, and has gained plenty of experience and knowledge about cars, motorbikes, boats, the sea and weather.

## Emma, age 16 months

Emma's parents told me, "She has always has been a very easygoing baby, tender and kind. At home at the moment her favourite thing is to take everything out of the cupboards and to explore everything she can reach. She loves to climb on things and up and down the stairs." Her parents' first language is Spanish and they also speak fluent English. She sleeps and eats well and not only is she beginning to talk, saying quite a few words in Spanish, but she is also very good at signing if she wants something she cannot say the word for – such as if she is tired or wants to eat. "We started signing with her when she was about 5 months old and she uses it a lot now."

## The parents' perspective: choosing a nursery

Before her first birthday Emma's mother wanted to return to work, so she started to look for a childminder or a nursery. Living in an inner-city area, there seemed to be many different possibilities to choose from, but only one suited her parents' needs at the time they wanted her to start. She started two days a week two months ago in a local, community-run day nursery. Her parents are very happy with the nursery, which they feel is welcoming and friendly, and as it happens some of the staff speak Spanish too. "This is an added bonus although not why we chose this nursery, but we did feel that if Emma was upset then they could talk to her in her first language."

Before Emma started the key person gave her parents a form to complete about Emma and then discussed it in detail with them to ensure she knew all she needed to about Emma and her care routine. There were particular things her parents requested of the nursery, such as about her feeding, sleep and toileting routines. Emma settled well. Although the nursery provides a daily sheet of written information about Emma's toileting, feeding, sleeping and some activities, this is just a tick sheet. When they pick her up in the evening the staff always say that she has "been fine", but do not give them any details about what has been special about the day for Emma. As they feel she has settled well and there are no causes for concern, they are happy, but they would like to know a bit more.

## What have we found out?

Although Emma's parents are very happy with the nursery and Emma herself is very contented to be there, her parents wanted to have more detailed daily information about how Emma had been. Once the nursery realised this they addressed it. Emma's mother has become increasingly involved in supporting the nursery since this time and is now on the Parent Committee. Emma continues to enjoy her nursery experience.

### Activity

From the examples above, both sets of parents were very happy with their choice of care, but Emma's parents wanted a stronger partnership with the key person and other staff in the room, and to find out a bit more on a daily basis about what Emma had been doing.

Find out the sort of detail your setting gives to the parents about what the children or babies have been doing during the day. Do you think parents find this useful? How can you find out?

# What the experts say
## Why partnership with parents matters

A major project called Effective Provision of Preschool Education (EPPE) headed by Professor Kathy Sylva of Oxford University and colleagues is one of the largest long-term research studies on the impact of early years provision in Europe. The research began in 1997 to find out whether preschool provision for children between the ages of 3 and 5 years has any impact on children's achievements by the age of 5, and, if so, the characteristics of the provision that seemed to make a difference. The research studied 3,000 children who attended different types of settings: playgroups, nursery classes in primary schools, maintained nursery schools, day care settings and integrated care and education settings (now called Children's Centres).

One of the aspects of provision the project researched was the effectiveness of partnerships with parents.

*"The most effective settings shared child-related information between parents and staff, and parents were often involved in decision making about their child's learning programme. There were more intellectual gains for children in centres that encouraged high levels of parental involvement."*

(Sylva *et al.*, 2004)

They also researched the effect of what parents did with their 3- and 4-year-old children at home to support their learning.

*"The home learning environment has a greater influence on a child's intellectual and social development than parental occupation, education or income. What parents do is more important than who they are, and a home learning environment that is supportive of learning can counteract the effects of disadvantage in the early years."*

(Melhuish *et al.*, 2008)

The research has had a huge impact on government policy in relation to early years, and it continues to research the same sample of children to see whether the effect of their preschool education is still evident through their school years. So far there have been reports on the children at age 5, 7, 11 and 14 years.

## Research on the impact of parental involvement in schools

In 2003 Charles Desforges, who is well known for his educational research about teaching and learning, and his colleague, Alberto Abouchaar, carried out a very useful review of research into partnership with parents and parental involvement in schools, entitled, *The Impact of Parental Involvement, Parental Support and Family Education on Pupil Achievement and Adjustment: A Literature Review.* (Desforges and Abouchaar, 2003). Although the report involved mainly school education, the findings are still important to those involved in working in the early years.

Desforges and Abouchaar looked at research that examined what parents did at home that involved them in their children's learning, as well as their participation with the school through events, helping in the classroom, and so on. They found that the most influential factor affecting children's achievements in school was what parents did at home with their children, such as providing a secure and stable environment, intellectual stimulation, helping the children see themselves as learners, providing opportunities for discussion and having positive social values and high aspirations. They also looked at parental involvement such as participating in school events, the classroom and even being involved as a school governor. Their summary showed that children whose parents take an active interest in their schooling make greater progress than other children, and in schools with similar intakes of children it was those where partnerships with parents were strongest that the children did best.

So to provide the best for the children in the early years, including in school nursery and reception classes, it is most likely that the findings would be similar. Finding out what parents do with their children at home and supporting parents by using our expertise in child development and how children learn is therefore very important.

## Effective practice:
## What do we need to do?

Effective partnership means that parents can be involved as partners in all aspects of the life of a setting. There is not room in this book to look at *everything* parents could be involved in, so the diagram below only shows the aspects that are covered. Being able to communicate well with parents in a friendly, clear and confident way is the key to success.

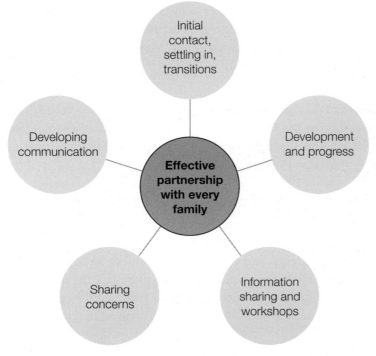

**Figure 5.4** Ways of involving parents in the life of a setting

## Initial contact and settling children in

### Creating a welcoming atmosphere

- Ensure parents feel welcome at all times. It is easy to assume we have created a welcoming atmosphere, but is it welcoming to *all* parents? Displays in your entrance about some of the learning experiences you provide will help, especially photographs with short, simple captions. Most of all, it is the smile and welcome that parents, children and visitors receive from you that makes the difference.

### Informing parents about your setting

- Have a small photo album or small photo booklets showing some of the activities, learning experiences and routines for parents to see when they first visit before the child starts. They will not be able to see

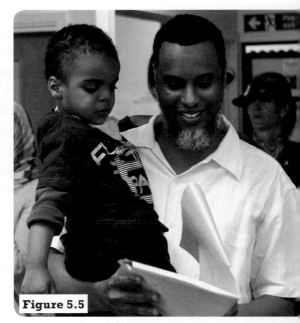

**Figure 5.5**

everything on a short visit, so these are really helpful for the parent and the child to look at and talk about. Keep it simple and child-friendly for sharing with the child. Remember that not everyone will understand things such as messy play as you do: explaining what is going on in the photos is important.

### Activity

Collect some photos of your setting that you think best illustrate what you do in your setting. Put these together into a small booklet, with a short sentence on each page to go along with the photo, which can be read to the child – for example, "When you come to our nursery you can play in the sandpit, play outside in the den or play with blocks."

### Settling-in procedures

- Provide some general information for parents outlining what they should expect when settling in their child. You may be the first person the parent has ever left their child with, so the parent is settling in as well as the child! It is the way you communicate at this sensitive time that makes all the difference. Good communication is not just about being able to tell parents what you feel they need to know, it is also about being a good listener, taking on board what parents tell you. Enable parents to express their hopes, fears and aspirations about their children.

### Home visits

- Many settings are able to set up home visits for children just before they start. Not all parents will want one and the purpose of them needs to be made very clear: to begin to get to know the child where he or she feels most at ease – at home. The children may have visited your setting already, but where home visits are possible, they can have real benefits in building positive relationships and settling children in. Usually two members of staff go on the home visit, the key person to play with and get to know the child, and another member of staff who can spend time talking with the parents about the setting and about their child. Taking small photo albums or booklets of your setting with you can really help.

### Finding out about the child before he or she begins

■ Have a list of questions to ask parents before the child starts. This can be written as a questionnaire that parents can complete at home or could be completed by parents and the key person together in the setting. A questionnaire is useful, but the conversation between staff and parents is vital too. A model list of questions is shown below.

**Child's name:** ............................................................ **Date of birth:** ................................................................

**Date of entry:** ....................................................... **Age at entry:** ................................................................

**Languages spoken at home:** .............................................................................................

Names of other family members and other significant people close to child:

Any previous experience of being cared for outside the home or by carers other than parents/ principal carers:

Does your child have any particular play interests at the moment, or particular toys he or she likes to play with?

What other sorts of things does your child show interest in or talk about?

How does your child respond to situations and people who are new to him or her?

Is your child used to being with/playing with other children and does he or she enjoy this?

Do you think your child's communication and language development is what you would expect for his or her age?

Does your child enjoy books and listening to stories? Does he or she have any favourite rhymes, stories, DVDs or CDs?

Does your child enjoy and get involved in imaginative-type play and role play?

Does your child show interest in activities such as building or constructing, matching and counting?

If you have a garden that your child can play in or if you go to the park, what does your child like to do?

Do you feel your child's physical development is what you would expect for his or her age?

What do you expect your child will like about the nursery/playgroup/school?

Does your child have any particular fears, worries or dislikes we should know about?

Is there any more information you would like to know about the nursery/playgroup/school and what your child will be doing?

Do you have any concerns or worries about your child's development?

Is there any other information you would like us to know in order to help your child settle and be happy?

*(Adapted from Hutchin, 2007)*

Remember, if you are unsure about something, for example, about a family's cultural or religious background, do not make assumptions. Find out from the parents themselves. Start from the point that every family is different and everyone needs equal respect.

## Activity

What kind of information do you as a practitioner need when a child or baby first starts with you? Make a list with other practitioners in your setting. Does your setting collect the information you all agree you need?

### Getting to know the children

■ Share your first observations of a new child with their parents as soon as you can. This will be important in helping parents feel at ease about leaving their child and helping you plan together for him or her. You will need to have some ideas of what you are looking for in the early days as the child is settling in, for example:

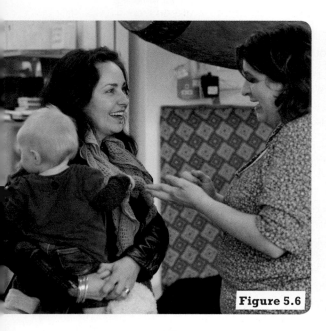

Figure 5.6

- How is the child responding to meeting/being with other children and unfamiliar adults?
- What makes the child feel most at ease?
- What is the child interested in exploring inside and outside?
- How is the child managing to express needs and feelings?

### Keeping in touch day to day

■ Ask the parents to let you know about anything they notice about their child at home during this settling-in period (such as being very tired). Make sure you have time with parents each day about the child's response to your setting, as well as discussing any other queries they may have.

## Sharing information about children's development and progress

### On a day-to-day basis

■ Make time on a daily basis for a two-way discussion between parents and the key person, sharing what the child has been doing both at home and in the setting.

### Meetings and reviews

■ Ensure there are procedures in place for regular discussions between key persons and parents, for example, at least every three months for 3–5-year-olds and more frequently for younger children and children with additional needs. This means a definite time is devoted to giving feedback to parents on their child's development, to ask parents about what the child is doing at home and to allow the parents to contribute their views about what the child is doing in the setting. Note down what parents say. Many settings have a form that they complete and parents sign.

### Involving parents in planning

■ Involve parents in discussions about possible next steps for their child during the regular review meetings. In this way parents can be involved in discussing how they may help the child at home as well as what will be planned in the setting.

# Information sharing workshops, programmes and celebrations

- Organise workshops meetings for parents to discuss various aspects of parenting, such as child development and play, areas of learning, managing behaviour, sleep and healthy diets. This is something that the EYFS encourages settings to do. Encourage parents to attend by:
  - choosing topics that parents want to know more about
  - choosing a time of day or day of the week that suits parents best
  - asking parents who you know will definitely be coming to invite others
  - making sure there is plenty of time for discussion and questions.
- Children's Centres usually have a wide range of workshops for parents to attend with their children, such as this song and rhyme session at Woodlands Park, which is run by one of the parents. The session became so popular with local parents that after a few weeks they had to run two sessions every week rather than one!

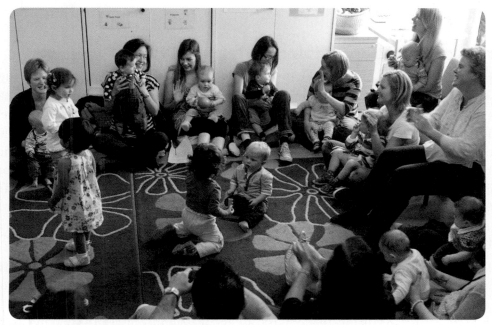

**Figure 5.7** A music and singing session at Woodlands Park

## Providing support to parents

- There are many specific programmes designed to help families who may be under stress or just in need of additional help for one reason or another. You may have heard of some of these, especially if you are involved with or work in a Children's Centre. There are some useful findings from these programmes as to what works well and some of the points discussed in this chapter have been shown to help, such as:
  - maintaining a friendly, trusting relationship
  - being accepting of all parents and treating all parents equally – not having negative views of some and being friends with others
  - taking parents' views into account and being a good listener
  - helping parents to find the advice they need.

### Celebrations and events

- Arrange social events and celebrations, as this is often the best way to get parents involved and, from this, to become involved in other things. Having fun together is so important and will build a community. The necessary fundraising events are likely to be so much more successful if everyone is having fun.

---

**Activity**

1  What happens in your setting to ensure a two-way partnership with parents?

2  Are there stronger relationships with some parents than others?

3  How are parents involved in your setting?

4  From the information in this chapter, what more do you think your setting could be doing?

---

## Sharing concerns and giving help and advice

Perhaps the hardest part of working with young children is sharing a concern you may have about a child's development, well-being or behaviour with their parents. But it is just as hard for the parent to share their concerns with you. Maintaining a good relationship when everyone is anxious is difficult. When concerns are expressed, allowing time, a confidential place to talk and good listening skills are particularly important. Note down the concerns raised and pass these on to your supervisors or manager. Make sure you know the proper procedure for your setting. Remember: the aim is not to be *friends* with the parents of the children in your care, but to be *friendly* at all times.

## Developing good communication skills

One of the most important aspects of developing a partnership with parents and building trusting relationships is your skills in communicating. Knowing the key skills of good conversation and being able to apply them will help to build your confidence.

- *Time:* Making time to talk together builds trust and reassurance, as well as making the parent feel really welcome. Sometimes a space away from the busy room in a nursery setting is necessary so that you are not interrupted, and for a childminder this may mean a meeting once the other children have gone home.

- *Listening:* Being an attentive listener is vital. For a new child you will want to ask some questions to find out all you can about him or her. But are you really able to listen to the answer? Research shows that in a conversation, only 7 per cent of what you communicate is the actual words you say. The rest of the communication comes from your tone of voice (38 per cent) and non-verbal gestures (55 per cent). Being an attentive listener means being aware of your non-verbal communication and tone of voice as well as the words used. Attentive listening helps the person speaking to you because you are making eye contact, showing interest in your facial expression and using gestures such as nodding.

- *Checking you have got it right*: Once the conversation is flowing, and without interrupting the flow, check every so often that you have understood it correctly – "So, I think you said she is ..." This gives a useful space for the parent to think if there is anything more they need to say, as well as checking you have got it right. This is invaluable if the parent is worried or wants to clarify something, and helps you both to order your thoughts if the conversation is becoming wide-ranging.
- *Asking questions*: You may need to ask more questions about the important things you still need to know about, but building up trust means listening more than asking questions, so limit your questions. The more open your questions can be, the better. Open questions are those that cannot be answered with one word, usually yes/no; instead, they often begin with "how?" or "why?"
- *Summarising*: At the end of a conversation it is important to summarise what has been said so that both of you are aware that the conversation is drawing to a close and what the main points made were. This is also an opportunity to decide on any matters to be dealt with, moving on to agreeing who will do what.
- *Giving information*: When you are giving information about the nursery or your care routines, many of the communication skills described above are needed. Make sure you are clear about what you want to say first, and ensure you give opportunities for the parent/carer to ask questions as necessary. Summarising at the end of each point is crucial – have you been understood? Finally, have you also taken on board the parent/carer's responses?

## Case study: Parental involvement at Fiveways Play Centre

Fiveways Play Centre is the voluntary-sector preschool discussed in the case study in Chapter 4. Parental involvement and working with other professionals, such as speech and language therapists and health visitors, are key strengths of the provision at Fiveways. Although it is run by a parent committee, the managers and staff are well aware that partnership with parents is always something that needs to be well thought out so every parent is involved.

They use a wealth of strategies to ensure that every parent is involved. These include:
- celebration events where parents bring in food they have cooked to share
- an illustrated booklet for parents, describing in photos exactly how each session works; this really helps the children understand what happens, as well as the parents
- regular newsletters to update parents since many are working
- regular open evenings for parents to talk to their child's key person and look at their child's learning journal; at the most recent evening the children each made their own individual invitation to their parents, which proved a highly successful strategy, drawing more parents to the meeting than ever before
- parents take the learning journals home after parents' evening, so that they can be shared with the family (they always come back again as parents are aware how important these are to the staff)
- a stay and play event for local parents with younger children is held twice a week, along with the occasional Saturday stay and play

- providing first-hand experiences for parents at some events, such as playing with play dough
- inviting specialists to present at events such as the AGM – for example, a dance and music specialist
- a regular survey of parents' views about the centre.

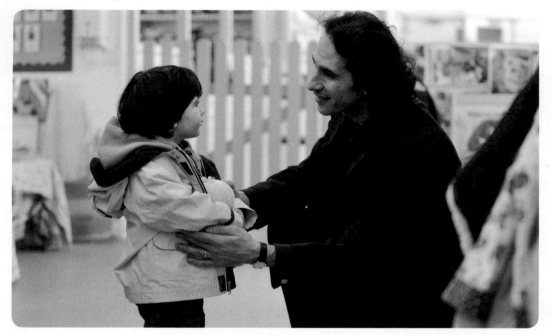

**Figure 5.8** Going home at the end of the day

## Chapter summary

This chapter will have helped you:
➤ recognise the importance of positive and honest relationships between a child's parents and practitioners
➤ develop your listening skills, understanding the importance of asking open questions to encourage genuine communication and a two-way partnership
➤ know about some of the research on why parental involvement in your setting is so important.

## Further reading and references

Bruce, T., Meggitt, C. and Grenier, J. (2010) *Childcare and Education*, Hodder Education, London

Desforges, C. and Abouchaar, A. (2003) *The Impact of Parental Involvement, Parental Support and Family Education on Pupil Achievements and Adjustment: A Literature Review*, Department for Education and Skills, London

Hutchin, V. (2007) *Supporting Every Child's Learning in the EYFS*, Hodder Education, London

National Strategies/DCSF, 'Inclusion Development Programme: Supporting Children with Behavioural, Emotional and Social Difficulties: Guidance for Practitioners in the Early Years Foundation Stage' (2010) National Strategies/Department for Children, Schools and Families, London

Ofsted (2007) 'The Foundation Stage: A Survey of 144 Settings', Department for Education and Skills, London

Sylva, K., Melhuish, E.C., Sammons, P., Siraj-Blatchford, I. and Taggart, B. (2007) *Effective Pre-school and Primary Education (EPPE 3–11) (2003–2008)*, Institute of Education, University of London

Tickell, C. (2011) *The Early Years: Foundations for Life, Health and Learning. An Independent Report on the Early Years Foundation Stage to Her Majesty's Government*, Annex 9, p.92. Available to download from: www.education.gov.uk

Walcot Foundation (2011) *P for Partnership: Practitioners Working in Partnership with Parents in the London Borough of Lambeth*, Early Education, London

## Useful websites

Early Home Learning Matters: www.earlyhomelearning.org.uk

Effective Pre-school and Primary Education (EPPE 3–11) (2003–2008): www.ioe.ac.uk/schools/ecpe/eppe

Family & Parenting Institute: www.familyandparenting.org

Louder than Words: Nonverbal Communication: www.minoritycareernet.com/newsltrs/95q3nonver.html

National Children's Bureau: www.ncb.org.uk

Parents, Early Years and Learning (PEAL): www.peal.org.uk

# **Section 2:** The characteristics of learning – how children learn

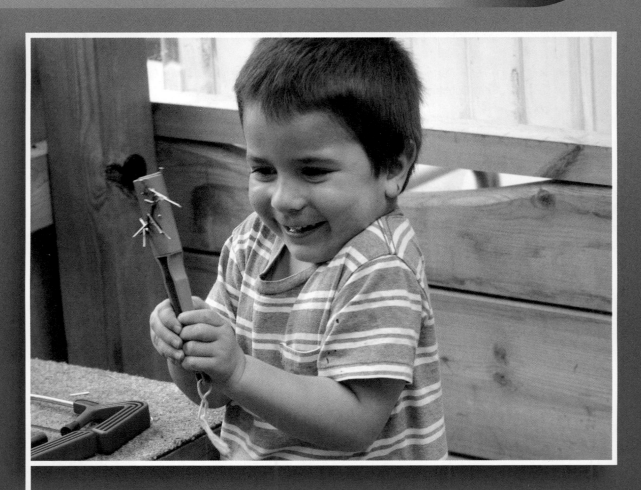

The revised EYFS has highlighted three "characteristics of effective learning", which describe the key ways that children learn:

➤ Playing and exploring (Chapter 6)
➤ Active learning (Chapter 7)
➤ Creating and thinking critically (Chapter 8).

These characteristics are about the processes of learning – in other words how children learn – and are formed from the first three commitments of the theme Learning and Development. They are lifelong characteristics that help us to be successful learners.

The chapters in this section take each of the characteristics in turn, explaining how practitioners can effectively help to facilitate children's learning and development, both through children's own self-chosen activities and play, and through adult-led activities and experiences.

## Chapter 6

# Playing and exploring

## In this chapter we will be looking at:

➤ the concepts of playing and exploring and why they are so important to children's learning and development

➤ some observations of children at play and analysing these to draw out the processes of learning that are taking place

➤ the views of experts who have helped us to understand play

➤ what we do to ensure our practice is effective in supporting children to learn and develop through playing and exploring.

## Introduction

Playing and exploring is the first of the three characteristics of effective learning highlighted in the EYFS 2012. Although we discussed this characteristic briefly in Chapter 4, we look at it here in greater detail. The photograph here shows a group of children: both boys and girls are playing in the home corner. At first glance they could be mistaken for playing together, but this is not strictly the case. What we see is different types of play going on. The two oldest children, both boys of just 3 years old, have a definite intention to play together, to create a pretend tea party. One girl asks to have some tea poured in her cup. The youngest child, age 19 months, had been deeply involved earlier in the day, exploring the resources,

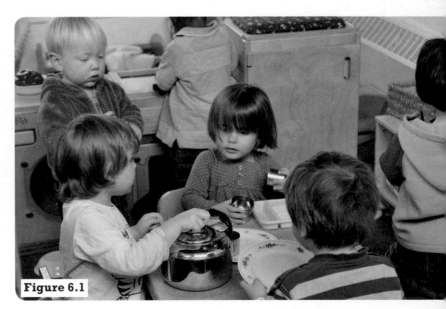

**Figure 6.1**

and now watches the others with interest. Another two children have their own play agendas, also exploratory. One is involved in playing at the kitchen sink and the other in exploring some of the resources on the shelves.

In one way or another they are all playing, whether it is exploratory play with the resources and equipment or pretend play in which a story is emerging through some children cooperating and developing this together. None of this would have happened in this way if the practitioners had not set up the home corner so that several children could choose to play here, following what interests them, using imagination and developing ideas. The open-ended nature of the resources provided has facilitated different kinds of play to suit the children, and was inclusive to all of them.

Those working in the early years are so lucky, not only to witness the remarkable development and learning that happens through play, but also to be supporting it. What a privilege to be involved at such a crucial time in the children's learning journey! The 'Early Years Learning Development: Literature Review', published in 2009, puts the importance of play and the role of practitioners in supporting it as one of its main findings: "Play is a prime context for development... there are now studies on different kinds of play, especially the ways it can be enriched by guiding, planning and resourcing on the part of staff in settings" (Evangelou *et al.*, 2009). This important research document, which formed part of the initial review of the 2008 EYFS, has helped to draw attention to this characteristic of learning in the 2012 EYFS.

## The EYFS characteristic of learning, Playing and exploring, tells us:

In the 2012 EYFS, as in the 2008 version, play is seen as vital to learning:

"Play is essential for children's development, building their confidence as they learn to explore, to think about problems, and relate to others."

(EYFS Statutory Framework, 2012)

And what is more, there is an in-built motivation to explore and to play: it seems to come naturally.

## What is this characteristic of learning about?

Playing and exploring is the first of the three characteristics of learning, because play and exploration enable children to become *fully engaged* in learning. "Play is an integrating mechanism. Play organises children's thinking, feelings, relationships and physical body so that everything comes together to support learning" (Bruce *et al.*, 2010).

The 2012 EYFS draws attention to three of the processes that form key components or aspects of what happens when children are playing and exploring:
1 **Finding out and exploring**
2 **Playing with what they know**
3 **Being willing to have a go.**

They are seen as important processes in children's learning, and reception teachers are asked to provide information to Year 1 teachers on what has worked best to support children to develop them. It is important for all practitioners to understand what they mean if we are going to be able to plan the appropriate support and assess its impact. In Chapter 4 we looked at the 'Play and exploration' commitment in the 2008 EYFS. Part of the commitment statement was that: "In their play children learn and develop at their highest level" (EYFS card 4.1). There is a great deal of research that establishes that play is essential to learning. Although children *can* learn and develop "at their highest level" through play, we need to make sure we are providing the best conditions for their play to flourish.

## 1. Finding out and exploring

There is a developmental sequence or pattern in the ways that babies, toddlers and young children play. The early part of the developmental sequence, up to around the age of 1 year, links very closely to the first of the three aspects of play highlighted in the EYFS Finding out and exploring. This element of play is often called exploratory play. Finding out and exploring results from children's "innate curiosity" and provides the experiences "from which children build concepts, test ideas and find out" (Tickell, 2011).

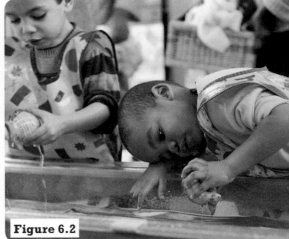

**Figure 6.2**

### At the beginning

To a baby, everything is new and needs to be explored. Babies begin to learn about the world around them by exploring and playing with objects through movement and all their senses, particularly their mouths. As they become mobile, they also want to explore every part of the space around them too. It is almost as if there are constant questions in their heads: "What is this?" and "What does this do?" followed by "What can I do with this?" As they do this they are in control of their own explorations, finding the method that suits their interests at the time.

Many researchers, such as Alison Gopnik and colleagues (1999), describe babies and toddlers as scientists who frequently repeat their tests and experiments to see what happens. This is their *exploratory play*: sometimes repeating the same actions time and again and at other times trying something new and different. Although this exploratory play is typical in babies, it continues into adulthood, and we as adults use this approach with things that are new to us (though we are unlikely to use our mouth or toes in the same way as babies do!).

### Supporting exploratory play

Giving young babies and toddlers predictable toys made of similar materials such as plastic limits their playful explorations. The richer the provision the better – for example, different textures, weights and materials – but it is essential that everything babies and toddlers come across is completely safe. This is where treasure baskets and heuristic play, first developed by Elinor Goldschmied and now used in many early years settings for babies, come into their own.

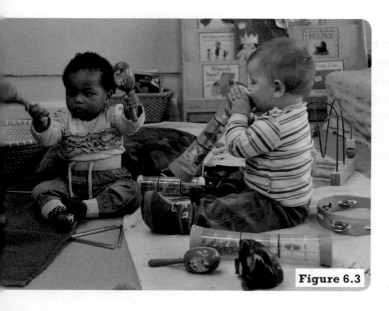

Treasure baskets and heuristic play are about providing natural objects and resources that are not toys for children of this age to explore. You can find out more about treasure baskets and heuristic play in Chapter 8.

In the photograph you can see two babies deeply involved in exploratory play. They are going through the sequence mentioned earlier, from "What is this?" to "what can I do with this?" The more opportunities babies, toddlers and young children are given to explore safely in their own ways, whether by banging and shaking, dropping objects on the floor, throwing or mouthing, the better it is for their learning and development. These are the early stages of problem solving and developing flexibility of thought.

**Figure 6.3**

In her book, *How Children Learn: The Characteristics of Effective Learning*, Nancy Stewart summarises some of the latest research on play and its potential impact on learning. She points out that "not all children have the same levels of exploratory play and these differences emerge very early in life" (Stewart, 2011, p.26). One piece of research showed that babies of 11–12 months who explored more "showed more successful and complex problem solving". These are important skills throughout life, so encouragement and support in the earliest years from parents, practitioners and professionals, by providing rich, safe provision in a safe environment, is important.

## Toddlers and the beginnings of imaginative play

Providing role play and imaginative play opportunities for toddlers is important. As babies become fully fledged toddlers a new kind of play develops, as they begin to imitate things they see others do, especially their parents and close adult carers. This imitative play is the early stages of imaginative and role play. At first it is a close imitation of actions, such as pretending to drink or feed a doll or teddy. The observation of William at 19 months in Chapter 3 shows him not only exploring "What can I do with this?" but also moving into the early stages of imaginative play as he holds the cup to the spout of the kettle.

## 2. Playing with what they know

The second process in Playing and exploring that is highlighted in the 2012 EYFS is: Playing with what they know, which can also be considered as play as an integrating mechanism. As the Tickell Review put it, this "... describes the importance of play as a context to bring together their current understandings, flexibly combining, refining and exploring their ideas in imaginative ways" (Tickell, 2011).

As they grow and develop, so do children's abilities to imagine. Their play develops from imitating to the world of imagination beyond the here and now. They are able to create imaginary scenes in their heads that they can then act out, using whatever is available to them. For example, the observation of Samira in Chapter 9, at age 2 years 8 months, shows her deeply involved in her imaginative world with a toy dog who is sick. Although playing on her own, she is also involving others, not in cooperative play, but as extras in her narrative (storyline). She *narrates* what she is doing to her key person and takes her medical equipment to check out some of the children, who easily accept this imaginary play. Her medical equipment consists simply of a pencil, which symbolises a syringe for injections. She is involved in what Tina Bruce calls free-flow play (Bruce, 1999).

As with Finding out and exploring, Using what they know in their play is a process that continues throughout childhood, becoming more sophisticated as children develop. However, not all children play imaginatively in this way for one reason or another, and as it is vital to development it is important that adults are on hand to help those who need additional support.

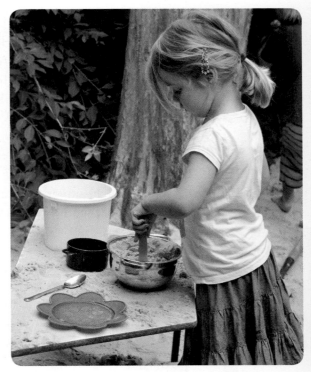

**Figure 6.4** Sand play can provide wonderful opportunities for being imaginative

### Activity

Can all children in your setting get involved in imaginative play? Think about the quieter children who may be shy of others: how are they being helped to join in? What about children who are not sure how to approach other children to get involved in play with them? How can you help?

## Development of cooperative play

Imaginative play develops further as imagination grows and children develop increasingly complex fantasies. The narratives (storylines) become more elaborate and children are usually very keen to involve others in their play. This is when cooperative play in a pair or small group comes into its own. But incorporating another child's viewpoint and wishes as well as one's own in imaginative play is not easy. As Gordon Wells states after analysing a vast amount of recorded evidence of children at play: "One of the striking characteristics of such play is how much of the time is spent in negotiating roles and appropriate actions, with the result – in some cases – that there is no time actually left to put the decisions into effect!" (Wells, 1987)

Learning to negotiate with each other is an important part of the play. Cooperative play enables children to explore a wide range of concepts and ideas, and generate their own problems to solve. Children continue to want to play alone for some of the time too. When they do this (and even in play with others) you will often hear them talking to themselves, giving a running commentary, narrating the storyline, as well as acting out the characters.

### Making rules

As you watch and become involved in children's fantasy and imaginative play, you will notice that as they take on a particular character or assign a character to another child or toy, they are making up rules as to what each character can do and how they are to behave. This rule-making is an integral part of the play, helping the children to cooperate and maintain the story. At any point the children can change their rules to take on another child's idea, keeping the play going or moving it in another direction.

### Being in control

Being in control is an important feature of all types of play and exploration. Children must remain in control of their play if it is to be useful to them in developing their skills and thought processes. As practitioners we need to begin by observing the play before joining in, not only to pick up children's particular interests so these can be followed up, but to work out how to enrich play to ensure learning continues. Adult support can prevent the play from becoming repetitive or stuck, but the children need to remain in control and the adult becomes a play partner, taking on a role allocated by the child. Children developing rules about what each character can or cannot do is an important part of being in control.

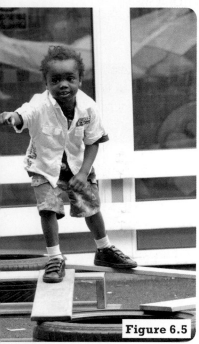

**Figure 6.5**

### Physical play

Physical play using the whole body is essential to children's all-round development and healthy growth. In the earliest stages of development, babies use movement to explore their surroundings, using their whole bodies. As children become more mobile they explore what their bodies can do – running, climbing, and so on – and they also incorporate their physicality into their play. Some play, such as play fighting or rough-and-tumble play, can seem as if it will turn into real aggression, but children need to experience this type of play to know the limits of their own skills, as well as the social boundaries imposed by others. Adult attention (without getting involved or taking over) is important to ensure it does not tip over into hurting each other.

## 3. Being willing to have a go

Being willing to have a go is about children developing positive dispositions (or habits of mind) towards themselves and their learning. These dispositions encourage them to have a go, initiate activities, challenge themselves and be willing to take risks and make mistakes. Play provides one of the best contexts for children to have a go. Every child comes to an early years setting with a different set of skills and amount of confidence, but whatever their starting point, play helps them gain confidence and awareness of their own skills, and capabilities. This is because play is not for real, and the children can decide to move in and out of play at any point or repeat it as much as they like. Play helps them build that essential can-do attitude.

Play provides children with the opportunity to:
- try out what it might feel like to be another person (mother, father, baby, brother, sister) or another creature (a dog, cat, crocodile, and so on)

- make decisions and choices and try out what it is like to be in control
- practise existing skills and knowledge in new ways
- apply skills and knowledge that are in the process of being learned and developed
- learn to negotiate and try out new ways of relating to others
- manage feelings that may be frightening or enjoyable
- devise problems and be the one who solves them
- put developing language and communication skills to new uses.

All of the opportunities listed build on children's social and emotional development and levels of confidence, as well as what they already know and can do. Make sure children are supported to do these things through their play by providing:

- a rich and stimulating environment that builds on their interests
- adults who are aware of their play and on hand to support it without taking over.

## Activity

1 Choose a child in your group to observe and watch them playing for a few minutes. Take notes on what you see and a photograph or two to remind you of interesting aspects of the play. (You could use the camera's video function rather than write notes, but you will need to make time to look at the video to analyse it.)

2 Analyse the play using the list of opportunities provided through play described above. How many opportunities do you think this play provided? Is there evidence of how the child or children were: finding out and exploring, using what they know in their play and being willing to have a go?

## Looking at children: What do we see?

### Samira, age 2 years 8 months

Samira is in the home corner trying on dresses, hats and bags. She is with Poppy. She tells Poppy that she likes going to parties with aeroplanes and trains. She goes to the construction area and takes some large blocks out, saying to the others around: "I'm building an aeroplane to go on holiday." Poppy joins her and together they build another aeroplane, this time with small attribute blocks. Samira begins the countdown for her journey: "5, 4, 3, 2, 1," then says, "Oh dear, my aeroplane can't fly because it needs petrol!" She pretends to fill up with petrol while saying, "We're going to be late for the cinema!" She asks Poppy to come with her to the "Cinema, in England". Poppy sits next to her and the plane takes off. Samira is the pilot and holds an arch-shape block for the steering wheel.

### What have we found out?

Samira is not yet 3 years, but is deeply involved in imagining, using props to support the play. The storyline or narrative is very much hers, but she is able to maintain the interest and involvement of Poppy, who is a similar age. As she plays, Samira is using what she knows and is willing to have a go. She knows the attributes of the blocks well and finds the shape she needs to symbolise the steering wheel. The play gives her an opportunity to play at being in control (of the aeroplane), develop her confidence, enabling her to have a go, use her knowledge of place to name where she is going and what she is going to do. In this episode of play, Samira followed her own ideas, sustained the play, stayed in control while accommodating another child in her play (social development), and solved a pretend but important problem (no petrol).

### Zein, age 3 years 11 months

Zein and two other boys have just decided to go outside, but stop off at the block play area on the way. They begin to build individually, but the activity turns out to be more about talking about what they might build than actually constructing. Zein says he is going to make Batman's car, then changes this idea to Ironman. The three boys start telling each other that they have Spiderman socks on and each starts to show their socks to the others. Soon they get their coats and go outside.

The three boys are running fast up and down one side of the area, sometimes running around the perimeter of the whole outdoor area. Occasionally they slow down to look around or catch their breath. There are now four boys together; two of them are Ironman and two are Spiderman. They stop to plan the play. One boy has gloves on and Zein negotiates to borrow first one (covering the hands if you are either Spiderman or Ironman is important!) and then both. "Just for five minutes," says Zein. "I've got two gloves now." The boys then discuss who is going to be the baddie. As they are all superheroes, no one is willing to become the baddie. The boys move towards the wheel toys and wait for a turn.

### What have we found out?

Superhero play, coming from films and cartoons, is important to these boys, as to many others. The nursery school is providing these children with a breadth of experience across all areas of learning, but is fully aware that being superheroes is their passion. They enable children to play in this way, making sure they are fully aware of the rules, such as not interrupting other children's play. Zein is able to use what he knows in his play (for example, that gloves are important to superheroes, whose covered hands usually have special powers), and in attempting to develop the play he is willing to have a go at assigning roles. The episode soon fizzles out as the storyline has not been developed very far. It is more about being the character than developing a story. Not only is the play physical, allowing the children to develop their large

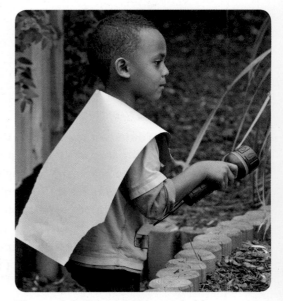

**Figure 6.6** This child has made his own cape for superhero play

muscles, but it is also very much about developing relationships and negotiating with each other. The school has also helped Zein to develop other interests too, for example, drawing and writing, interest in mini beasts and in books and stories that involve, like superhero play, elements of good and bad, and model clever ways of being in control, such as *The Gruffalo* by Julia Donaldson.

## Activity

### Superhero play and physical play

1  What are your feelings about allowing children to be involved in superhero play and very active physical play?
2  Should it be discouraged or should practitioners become involved in supporting the play?
3  What is the policy in your setting?
4  Check out what your colleagues feel about it. What about the parents?

## What the experts say
### Understanding the importance of play

Tina Bruce's work on play over the last 30 or so years has been very significant for early years practitioners and other professionals within the early childhood sector, not just across the UK but throughout the world. Probably her most well-known book about play for practitioners is *Learning Through Play: Babies, Toddlers and the Foundation Years* (Bruce, 2011). The book is very accessible and is quoted, for example, in Effective Practice in the 2008 EYFS. Bruce provides a very useful analysis of play and how it should be supported: "Play creates an attitude of mind which brings deep involvement in learning, fosters the desire to learn and to be an adventurous learner." She also highlights how play helps children to develop abstract ideas.

Bruce's first book specifically about play was *Time to Play in Early Childhood Education* (1991). In this she points out that many things that are called play may be things with a playful element but are not strictly play. She develops her theory about what she calls free-flow play (imaginative, creative play that flows freely from one thing to another) and its importance to learning. She sees free-flow play as part of a "network of related processes" that develop alongside the play, such as representation, humour and games. She develops a formula for free-flow play that demonstrates what is taking place when children's play is enabled to flow freely:

| Free-flow play | = | wallowing in ideas, feelings and relationships | + | application of developed competence, mastery and control |
|---|---|---|---|---|

Bruce also developed 12 features of play, which have been widely used by practitioners in defining rich play that engenders learning. Where at least seven of these features are visible when play is observed, the likelihood is that, the play will be rich in learning.

## Vivian Gussin Paley: Observing and analysing fantasy play

Vivian Gussin Paley is an American nursery teacher, now in her eighties, whose research throughout her career has been her own early years class and her own teaching. Paley's research develops from her daily tape recordings of the children at play, as well as her discussions with them and what takes place at storytime. Every evening she listens, transcribes and analyses her tapes of the day. Through this method she has developed wonderful deep insights into the world of early childhood and the overwhelming importance of fantasy play and stories as mechanisms for development and learning. In one of her early books, *Wally's Stories* (1981), she talks about her reasons for taping in the early stages of her career, which were to try "… to determine why some discussions zoomed ahead in an easy flow of ideas and others plodded to a halt" (Paley, 1981). She soon worked out that the better she listened to the children and let them express their ideas, the better the discussions.

To Vivian Gussin Paley fantasy play is "mankind's oldest and best loved learning tool". She believes that "Fantasy play, rather than being a distraction, helps children achieve the goal of having an open mind." "There is no activity children are better prepared for than fantasy play. Nothing is more dependable and risk-free, and the dangers are only pretend" (Paley, 2004). She helps the reader understand the overwhelming concerns for 3- to 5-year-olds, such as friendships, fairness and fears, and especially how fantasy play helps children to manage their feelings and feel in control among the complexities of the human world around them. She is always respectful of all the children she writes about and shows us their ability to think critically and to reason from a very young age.

An innovative element of her practice has been her story table, available every day for the children to come to her to dictate their own stories, which she scribes. At storytime the children then act out their own stories to the others. The stories are usually based on their fantasy play themes, as these are so significant to them.

Paley is a prolific writer and her very readable books are full of clear perceptions about early childhood and, most importantly, the role of the practitioner ("teacher") in supporting development and learning.

# Effective practice:
## What do we need to do?

How can we best support children's play and explorations? Playing and exploring are essential vehicles through which children learn. We provide the rich opportunities and the provocations for the play, and we also need to provide the sensitive encouragement and support. So, how do we do this?

Everything described so far in this chapter, including what the experts say, tells us that play and exploration:
- are chosen by the child – we cannot make them play or tell them how to explore, although we can encourage them
- are best when they flow freely and follow the direction set by the child.

It is not play unless the child is in control of the play agenda, the storyline and the rules of engagement. We cannot plan for a particular outcome to result from play, but it is very important that we plan to ensure that there are many opportunities for children to play, by:
- observing children and talking with parents to find out about the children's particular play interests and the ideas they are currently exploring
- providing interesting resources, interesting environments and plenty of time to play
- being on hand to support the play as a play partner: perhaps to support a child who is unsure how to join in, or a child with additional needs, or because children invited you in.

This will help ensure that the play is purposeful.

### Begin with children's interests
- Provide rich play environments that build on children's interests. At first, when children are new to the setting or group, you will need to find out from parents about the things the child is likely to be interested in, but as you get to know the child better, your observations will show his or her particular interests. It is important to remember that children will share interests, so catering for the interests of one child means catering often, but not always, for many.

### Sometimes, get involved
- Be on hand to get involved with children in their play and their explorations. Take your cue from the children.
- Become involved as a play partner, taking on the role that the children suggest and being prepared to take instructions from the children.

## Time to reflect: to get involved or not?

The *richest* play often happens between pairs and small groups of children, uninterrupted, with no direct adult involvement. The story flows seamlessly from one thing to another as children negotiate with each other, adding to and changing their story. When you see this happen, do not interrupt or get involved. Listening in and keeping an eye out can reveal the power of play to children's learning.

At other times your involvement, so long as it is *sensitive* and *the children remain in control*, can be one of the most effective ways of extending children's learning. Once involved in the play you can ask 'I'm not sure what to do – can you tell me?', or if appropriate, 'Where are we going?', 'How will we get there?' or you might act surprised by the price of goods in the pretend shop. In this way new vocabulary and language can also be introduced within the context of playing a part in the play.

### Involve parents

- Involve parents, not only by finding out about children's interests and types of play at home, but also informing them about the importance of play and the various ways in which play supports learning.
- Let them know about the kind of play their children are pursuing daily in the setting.

### Finding out and exploring

- Provide plenty of interesting opportunities and experiences for the children to explore using all their senses, including the environment inside and outside.
- Be sensitive. Always watch for a few minutes before you join in so that you do not cut across children's particular interests and so that they can keep involved and focused. Bear in mind that sometimes it may be better not to join in.
- Be on hand to talk with the children about their play. For older children this may be asking open questions about what they are doing or have been doing, showing that you are interested. For babies and toddlers and children who are less verbally advanced, or are new to learning English, you may be describing in simple language what you see them do.

### Playing with what they know

- Observe children at play so that you know whether your play provision is rich enough and encourages children to get the best from their play. Remember that play can take place anywhere. A rich environment for children's imaginative play will mean that the potential for imagination to flourish is in every aspect of your provision.
- Ensure there is plenty of time for children to be involved in play. More complex play, such as cooperative play in a group, requires time to get going. Not only does this mean making sure there is enough time allotted every day, but that a play scenario that children are developing and continue to enjoy is available day after day, with practitioners refreshing the environment and adding new resources in discussion with the children.

- Add play possibilities that are new and different, beyond the children's own experiences, which will act as provocations for new interests and new learning. Adult-led activities are important in helping to develop children's knowledge, skills and understanding, which they will then be able to use in their play – for example, an imaginative story or information book will fire their imaginations. An outing to introduce the children to the fire station or the local hairdresser's, for example, will be invaluable. Ensure the children decide with you the play props they want and how to set up the environment.
- Set up any new role-play scenario *with* the children. Evaluate it regularly to ensure this is sparking off new interests for the children. If not, decide whether it is the idea that is not working or if the provision is in the wrong place or needs more inspiring resources.

## Being willing to have a go

- Encourage children to have a go. This may mean getting involved in having a go yourself first if it is play that some children may be unsure of, such as clay or block play.
- Support children to develop confidence. Not all children are confident to play. Coming to a setting may be the first opportunity that a child has had to play with other children for any length of time. They may also be unsure about what to do and what is expected of them. Some children are unsure how to get involved with others – see Chapter 9 for more information. It is important to support children with additional needs in joining others in play appropriate to their needs.
- Ensure parents are fully aware about providing children with the right clothing so that they can play outside in all weathers and get messy.

## Chapter summary

This chapter will have helped you:
➤ understand more about why playing and exploring are such vital processes in children's learning and development
➤ find out more about the three aspects that the EYFS highlights in this characteristic of learning, with the help of observations of children
➤ become familiar with the work of two important experts in theories and research on play.

## Further reading and references

Bruce, T. (2011) *Learning Through Play: For babies, toddlers and young children*, Hodder Education, London

Bruce, T., Meggitt, C. and Grenier, J. (2010) *Child Care and Education*, Hodder Education, London

Evangelou, M., Sylva, K., Kyriacou, M., Wild, M. and Glenny, G. (2009) 'Early Years Learning and Development: Literature Review', DCSF Research Report RR176. Available to download from: www.education.gov.uk/publications/RSG/publicationDetail/Page1/DCSF-RR176

Paley, V.G. (1981) *Wally's Stories: Conversations in the Kindergarten*, Harvard University Press

Paley, V.G. (2004) *A Child's Work: The Importance of Fantasy Play*, University of Chicago Press

Stewart, N. (2011) *How Children Learn: The Characteristics of Effective Learning*, Early Education (The British Association for Early Childhood), London

Tickell, C. (2011) *The Early Years: Foundations for Life, Health and Learning. An Independent Report on the Early Years Foundation Stage to Her Majesty's Government*, Annex 9, p.92. Available to download from: www.education.gov.uk

Vygotsky, L. (1978) *Mind in Society*, Harvard University Press

Wells, G. (1987) *The Meaning Makers: Children Learning Language and Using Language to Learn*, Hodder Arnold, London

## Useful websites

Children's play information service: www.ncb.org.uk/cpis

Play England: www.playengland.org.uk/

# Chapter 7

# Active learning

## In this chapter we will be looking at:

➤ the meaning of active learning and how practitioners support this through actively engaging in play, self-chosen activities and appropriate adult-led activities

➤ some observations of children actively learning

➤ the views of experts who have helped us to understand the importance of motivation and active learning

➤ how we can ensure our practice is effective in supporting children's motivation to explore and learn.

## Introduction

Active learning is the second of the three characteristics of effective learning highlighted in the EYFS 2012. Although we briefly discussed this characteristic in Chapter 4, this chapter tells you more about it.

Tobi and Frankie are nearly 5 years old. Tobi often chooses to build with the blocks, both inside and outside. Today Tobi and Frankie are both highly involved in creating a long, snaking pathway from the bottom of the slide, around a large part of the outdoor area and back to the climbing frame. The idea for this came from Tobi, but Frankie is a very willing and highly motivated partner. They have used everything suitable to hand: all the hollow blocks, planks balanced on crates and a moveable tunnel to crawl through. Once completed, they run round on it several times. They have created a rule for themselves and a special challenge – not to put feet on the ground at any time. Many other children join in. They have not all taken on board Tobi and Frankie's game, so some have different ideas and want the end of the path to be elsewhere. However, as others dismantle it, Tobi and Frankie patiently mend their pathway again. The game continues for a considerable length of time until tidy-up time.

Tobi's ideas and skills in building and constructing have developed to a sophisticated level because of his motivation to pursue a special interest – block play – using the wonderful open-ended provision. The boys' creation has a purpose: to move around it without stepping on the ground, and others enjoy this challenge too. This is active learning. Although there are many physical aspects to this self-chosen activity, and its purpose presents a physical challenge, active learning is about having an idea and being able to carry it out – it is more about being *mentally* active than physically active.

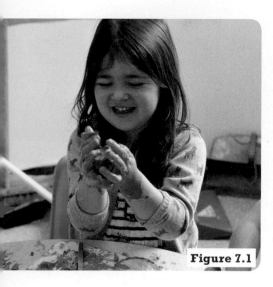

Figure 7.1

## The EYFS characteristic of learning, Active learning, tells us:

Active learning is closely associated with *motivation*, as the Tickell Review put it:

*"This strand highlights key characteristics which arise from intrinsic motivation to achieve mastery – to experience competence, understanding and autonomy"*

(Tickell, 2011)

Active learning is the second of the three characteristics of learning and, like the other two, reception teachers are asked to complete information on how each child makes use of this in assessments for the EYFS Profile.

## What is this characteristic of learning about?

## The EYFS 2008 commitment Active learning is discussed in Chapter 4 and states that:

*"Active learning involves other people, objects, ideas and events that engage and involve children for sustained periods."*

(EYFS card 4.2)

The children described in the Introduction to this chapter, who are nearly 5 years, are engaged and involved in their activity for a sustained period. The activity is self-chosen and carried out without adult involvement, but the adults created the context and the environment in which the boys could implement their own plans and ideas, thereby encouraging them to develop their skills.

The EYFS 2012 highlights three components or aspects of what children are doing when they are engaged in active learning. These are:

1 **Being involved and concentrating**
2 **Keeping on trying**
3 **Enjoying achieving what they set out to do.**

Children learn through actively investigating the world around them. There is an inner drive to be actively learning in this way from birth onwards and it is not specific to children in their earliest years, but continues throughout life if we foster it. To foster it, parents and practitioners need to make the conditions right for children to remain self-motivated and enjoy the challenge of learning. The dispositions and attitudes that children need to make this happen must be established early on in life if they are to be confident to have a go and develop a can-do approach to things they encounter. The role adults play in supporting children is important – we can encourage and facilitate active learning, or, unintentionally, we can act as a block on it.

# 1. Being involved and concentrating

Being involved begins with finding something interesting and intriguing enough to want to be involved. Motivation is key to concentrating on something, but it is highly individual. What motivates one person will not be the same as what motivates another. The Tickell Review talks about "the intensity of attention" children may give when "following a line of interest". When a baby, child or adult is deeply involved and concentrating it is likely that they are involved in deep-level learning and it is this deep-level learning, that we should all be aiming for. The 'Early Years Learning and Development: Literature Review' stated that in supporting children's thinking, "it is more important to aim at depth and not breadth. Deep understanding is more important than superficial coverage" (Evangelou *et al.*, 2009). A whole range of factors can motivate us.

Ferre Laevers (see What the experts say, later in this chapter) believes that the greater the level of involvement in an activity, the more likely it is that children will be involved in deep-level learning. It involves an element of challenge – pushing ourselves beyond the skills and understanding we have now towards something new. It allows us to puzzle something out so that we change the way we think about it, grasp a new idea or grapple with a new skill.

Being deeply involved and concentrating means that babies, children or adults are likely to block out interruptions and remain concentrating on the task in hand. We can actually see this as it takes place, and Ferre Laevers has developed a useful scale for measuring a child's involvement. But what sort of things do children concentrate on and get involved in? Research shows that when children are able to make their own choices, follow their own train of thought and make use of their natural curiosity, they are much more likely to become deeply involved and concentrate. This is why playing and exploring are so motivating for children and why child-initiated activities are so important. The motivation to become involved is not imposed from the outside but comes from within the child – this is intrinsic motivation.

## How do we help?

This type of learning has implications for practitioners. The EYFS asks that practitioners provide a balance of child-initiated and adult-led activities, because *both* are important in supporting learning. If being involved and concentrating leads to the kind of learning that we want all children to participate in, and it works best if it is the child's choice, how do we support it? What about the adult-led activities we also need to provide?

For *child-initiated activities* we need to ensure that the learning environment is stimulating, with novel as well as familiar things to explore, and that children's particular interests are catered for. Active learning is about the process of learning, not about an outcome or end product. As Nancy Stewart says, "Choice, time and space, freedom to follow ideas without anxiety about an end product" (2011). The choice, however, is the child's; adults need to be on hand though, encouraging children to explore further and try things out so that they can get deeply involved.

*Adult-led activities* will support learning by ensuring that any planned activity is based on the sorts of things that children will be interested in. Planned adult-led activities are not suitable for babies or young toddlers as they need time and space to explore, and plenty of attention from adults around them about what they are showing interest in. But from 2 years upwards, as long as the activity is open-ended, with no pressure or expectation for a particular outcome or product, adult-led activities will provide new avenues and new interests for children to explore.

## Activity

### Being involved and concentrating in an adult-led activity

If you work with children over 2 years, ask a colleague to observe a planned activity that you have organised and are leading.

1 Ask your colleague to focus on whether the children are fully involved (see page 103). It is not about how well the children are carrying out the activity, but how motivated and interested they are in it.

2 Ask your colleague to give you feedback.

3 If any child was not showing signs of deep involvement, what could you do next time instead?

If you work with under-2s, watch children involved in self-chosen activities.

1 Could you see the same signs as described on page 103?

2 If not, how could you vary your environment and provision so that they could become deeply involved?

## 2. Keeping on trying

The next component of active learning, Keeping on trying, could be described as a disposition or habit of mind. This is all about persisting with an activity, puzzling out an idea or developing a new skill, even though it might be challenging and difficult. You can see it in babies as they learn to crawl or walk, trying time and time again until they master the skill. Once they have got the basics there is much more to learn, for instance, in crawling, going from sitting to crawling or how to turn round, so the persistence continues.

## Case study: Emma, age 23 months

Every time Emma saw a scooter or a child using one she would head towards it: her interest was very obvious. Then Emma was given a scooter. She loved it so much she even went to sleep holding it! When she was taken outside with the scooter she either walked backwards pulling it along or stood on it with both feet. Her parents and family friends began to show her how to put one foot on the scooter and the other on the ground. At first they pulled her along so she got the feeling of moving. Then, with encouragement, she gradually worked out how to push with one leg to get the scooter moving, slowly at first, with frequent small steps. Even though it was still easier to pull it along while walking backwards, Emma persisted in trying to scoot, and over the next few days, with a small amount of adult guidance and a lot of adult patience, Emma worked out for herself how to scoot. This is a complex skill – Emma was very aware that she needed to work at mastering the skill, but she persisted. This is active learning, involving a can-do attitude towards herself.

Do we see persistence in every child or do some appear to give up very easily and avoid challenge? Carol Dweck's research (see What the experts say, later in this chapter) helps us to understand why some children (and adults) might give up easily and others enjoy any challenge and persist at it. It is all about developing a positive disposition to ourselves as learners – what Carol Dweck calls a "growth mindset". Parents and practitioners need to help children to develop this growth mindset.

## Helping children to persist

*"The way we see ourselves is shaped by the messages we receive from the significant people in our lives. When we receive encouragement for our efforts and our ideas are valued, our feelings acknowledged and our discoveries recognised, we come to see the world as a safe place, and ourselves as competent and capable agents within it. These positive messages give us the confidence to take on the risks and challenges that all new learning brings."*

(National Strategies DCSF, 2007)

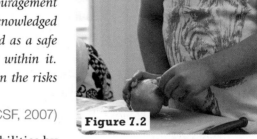

**Figure 7.2**

Inadvertently we can limit children's learning possibilities by squashing the drive to try out challenging things. If we always do things for children rather than letting them try themselves, we take away their independence and autonomy, making them more dependent on us. We need to encourage children by providing challenges that are achievable but not too easy. If something is likely to be too difficult we need to break it down into achievable steps. We also need to be very careful about how we give praise, so that the children see themselves as learners, not as clever or not clever. Talking with children about the learning processes they are going through and not the end product is very important and something we need to be doing regularly.

## Activity

Children explore and experiment very many times when they are learning something new. You may see them frequently repeating the same action and wonder why.

1 Observe a child absorbed in a child-initiated activity for a considerable length of time. Can you tell whether this was something within the child's comfort zone – something they could already do that they chose to repeat or something they were trying to master?

2 If it appears to be a skill or idea they already have, why do you think they may be repeating it?

# 3. Enjoying achieving what they set out to do

The final disposition for active learning sounds a bit clumsy: enjoying achieving what they set out to do, but it is about the enjoyment gained from achieving one's own intentions, or, as the Tickell Review puts it, "the satisfaction of meeting one's own goals... rather than relying on the approval of others" (Tickell, 2011). Active learning involves having some kind of goal in mind and we see this just as much in babies as in children and adults. Success in achieving it brings satisfaction. When watching babies and toddlers, however, we often have to observe carefully to work out what their goal is.

Nancy Stewart (2011) points out that "even though the concept of the self is still developing, very early in life we begin to identify and evaluate our own progress towards goals." We see this, for example, when babies and toddlers show delight in achieving the desired effect with a cause-and-effect toy, because they have made it happen themselves. Making and maintaining relationships with other children or with adults may often be the young child's self-chosen goal. Watching another child mastering a skill often sparks off a new interest in a child to achieve a similar goal. But whatever the goal is, when the goal is chosen by the child, he or she is fully motivated to keep on trying to achieve it.

There are different types of goals. There are those that come from within, linked to our internal intrinsic motivation, that are often to do with mastery of skills or understanding new ideas. Then there are those that result from an external incentive to do something – so achieving the goal means getting a particular reward. Exactly what motivates a young child may not always

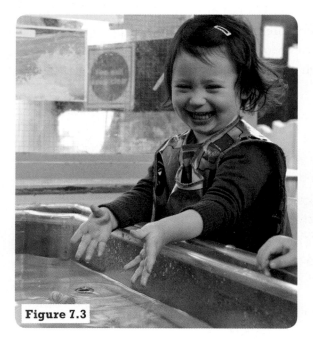

**Figure 7.3**

be clear, but it is an exciting process that pulls the child into deeper learning. The practitioner's role is to be aware and enable and encourage the self-motivation and deeper learning that is taking place. Positive relationships between significant adults and children will be a major source of support to children in achieving their own goals.

Of course, adults have goals for children to achieve too, such as what we want the children to be learning. Helping children to understand why we may have particular goals we want them to achieve is important if we want them to make it a goal of their own. If the goal becomes their own they will be motivated not by an external reward, but because they believe it is something they want or need to achieve. The commitment and determination will then come from within.

## Looking at children:
## What do we see?

### Alex, age 3 years 2 months, and Dylan, age 3 years 1 month

Alex and Dylan are sitting at the table in the home corner, playing with the kettle and tea set. The kettle has already been half filled by another child, with fruit and vegetables. The two boys pretend to pour tea into their cups, but the kettle is too heavy to pick up. As you can see from their expressions (in the following images), they are deeply involved and concentrating.

Another child nearby asks for a cup of tea, but their concentration is such that they do not hear. After a few minutes of her repeated questions she says to Alex, "I asked for some tea and you said no. Say no to Dylan too then ok!" Finally she gets her way and some pretend tea is poured for her (Figure 7.5).

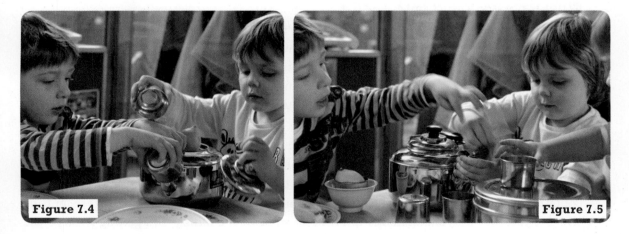

Figure 7.4

Figure 7.5

Alex is cramming the kettle full with more fruit and tries to fit the lid on, but he cannot. In his attempt to solve the problem (the fruit is real fruit!) he tries to take a bite out of the lemon, but in the end gives it to Dylan, who puts it in his tea cup. Now the lid can go on. Alex says the tea is "fruit salad tea". The play continues, with more children getting involved, but Alex and Dylan remain completely focused. Another child asks for tea. Alex hears this time, looks into the kettle and replies, "Okay, but it has practically all finished now!"

Once Alex resolved the problem of getting the lid on the kettle, both Alex and Dylan's attention turns to the small lid on the spout of the kettle (see Figure 7.6), but then Alex turns his attention back to the lemon again, for another attempt to fit it in the kettle (see Figure 7.7). They continue their deep involvement until it is tidy-up time.

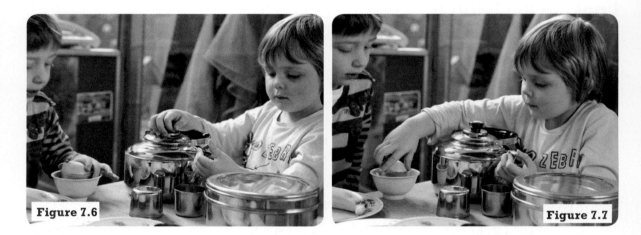

Figure 7.6    Figure 7.7

## What have we found out?

Both boys are deeply involved and concentrating, and with so many other children wanting to take part, this is not easy. With Alex, in particular, we can see how he keeps on trying: attempting to solve the problem of filling the kettle with all the fruit, but also in staying in control of the fruit salad tea he has decided to make, while maintaining relationships with others. Both Alex and Dylan show obvious signs of satisfaction about their involvement.

## Poppy, age 2 years 7 months

Baking with the 2-year-olds in this Children's Centre is a regular adult-led activity. The member of staff who is leading the activity informs the children of what they will be making and how. Poppy has her turn and attempts to stir the sugar and margarine. She sighs as she does so, putting all her effort into it as she manages to break up some of the lumps. "It's getting sugary," she says. She picks up a large lump of margarine and laughs, showing it to all the others. "Eurrgh," she says. She passes on the bowl to the next child when asked to. When she sees another child struggling, she says, "I'll show you," moving to take the spoon, but when asked to let the other child try, she does so. She helps to beat the egg and adds it to the mixture, saying, "We have to put in the flour now," remembering this from another occasion when she made cakes.

## What have we found out?

There is one bowl and part of the aim of the activity is to support children in taking turns in a communal activity. This was an adult-led activity. Poppy remained focused and stayed with the task because she wanted to be involved. She was able to remain fully involved and concentrating until the cake-making was completed. As this is a communal cooking activity she has to wait her turn, but she continues to focus on the tasks in hand. Her comments show how engaged she was and how she can apply her knowledge.

## What the experts say
## Being involved and concentrating

In talking about active learning and especially being involved and concentrating, the Tickell Review made reference to the work of Professor Ferre Laevers and his concept of deep-level learning (Tickell, 2011). We have already discussed his work on well-being in Chapter 1. We now look at his work on involvement and deep-level learning.

### The concept of involvement

Professor Laevers has been working on the concept of involvement since the 1970s. His work has been welcomed by practitioners across the UK and he is frequently invited to talk about his work. Ferre Laevers believes that when children are deeply involved in what they are doing, significant, *deep-level learning* is taking place: "… an involved person is driven by his exploratory need which puts him in a state of mind favourable for deep-level learning" (Laevers, 1994). As we have seen already, involvement is related to children's innate or intrinsic motivation and positive dispositions to what they are doing. This is how he describes the concept of involvement:

*"When children are concentrated* [sic] *and focused, interested, motivated, fascinated, mentally active, fully experiencing sensations and meanings, enjoying the satisfaction of the exploratory drive, operating at the very limits of their capabilities, we know that deep-level learning is taking place. If deep-level learning is taking place, a person is operating at the limits of their 'zone of proximal development'."*

(Laevers, 2002)

As we saw in Chapter 4, the term zone of proximal development came from Vygotsky and simply means that a person is challenging themselves at the upper limit of what they know and can do.

It is deep-level learning in young children that will have a lasting effect and practitioners can either enhance or impede it. As Laevers says: "If we want deep-level learning we cannot do without involvement" (Laevers, 2000). Increasing the levels of both well-being (discussed in Chapter 1) and involvement will enhance learning.

Laevers has devised systems for observing involvement as well as emotional well-being. His Leuven Involvement Scales have become a powerful evaluation tool, with a five-point scale for early childhood settings and schools. He provides a description of what involvement looks like at each scale point, from the lowest level of involvement at point 1 to the highest level of involvement at point 5.

There is no need to write the observation down, but rather to use the scale immediately after each observation to grade the level of involvement. Observing several times means that you will see a child involved in a variety of activities, which will then show a more accurate pattern of their level of involvement rather than just a one-off observation. If the observations of the child show that child is generally at a low level of involvement, or their involvement is low in certain activities, then action must be taken to support the child. The Leuven Involvement Scales are used in the *Effective Early Learning Programme* (Pascal *et al.*, 1997, 2007), a comprehensive self-evaluation programme used in many early years settings and schools across Britain.

## Keeping on trying

### Carol Dweck: Mindsets and mastering new skills

Carol Dweck is an American professor of psychology whose work has been increasingly recognised internationally. Her research is all about why some people are motivated to take on difficult tasks, and therefore push and challenge themselves, and others appear to shy away from such challenges and only try things they know they will be successful at. Her theory is that our mindset – the views we have of ourselves as learners – has a huge influence on how we are as learners. Her most well-known book, *Mindset: The New Psychology of Success* (2007), outlines much of her research over more than 30 years, with different groups of children of all ages and with adults.

Children's views about themselves as learners begin to be formed at an early age. Carol Dweck shows that we develop a mindset that will either help us in our ability to learn or will hinder it. Her theory refers to two mindsets: the fixed mindset and the growth mindset.

Those with the fixed mindset believe that their abilities are fixed and cannot be changed. They have a tendency to always want to get things right, because if they do not, they will feel a failure. People with a fixed mindset are unlikely to want to take on challenges they are unsure of, preferring to be in the safety zone of what they know they can achieve. Dweck believes that "People are all born with a love of learning, but the fixed mindset can undo it" (Dweck, 2007).

Those with the growth mindset are excited by challenge – they push their own boundaries and if they meet an obstacle they want to find a way round it, to find another way to succeed. Their underlying belief about ability is that it is not fixed, but can grow and develop. Carol Dweck's many experiments, including with 4-year-olds, show that the way children deal with problems demonstrates their mindset. "As soon as children become able to evaluate themselves, some of them are afraid of challenges. They become afraid of not being smart" (Dweck, 2007).

### What messages are we giving children?

The great thing is that a mindset is not fixed for life: it can be changed with help. The way we as parents and practitioners talk with young children can make a big difference. Carol Dweck believes that part of the problem of the fixed mindset is the influence that adults' views have on the child. We often show these by the things we concentrate on, for example, having the best end product, rather than focusing on the processes involved in doing something. The messages we give are key:

*"It can be a fixed mindset message that says 'You have permanent traits and I'm judging them'. Or it can be a growth mindset message that says: 'You are a developing person and I am interested in your development'"*

(Dweck, 2007)

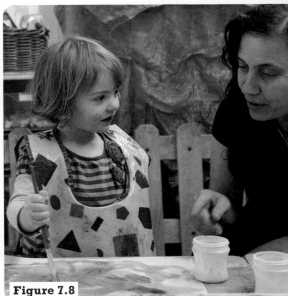

She points out how we do this by our casual comments to children.

Praising a child for their cleverness or intelligence may be done to try to boost confidence, but is more likely to result in the child developing a fixed mindset view where they will not want to keep on trying in the face of difficulties and problems, as they will feel put on the line and judged. However, praising children for their efforts or their choices, what they accomplish through practice, persistence and trying different strategies and approaches, will help to develop a growth mindset. It will also help to give children the chance to think about their own learning – an important strategy we discuss in the next chapter as we help children become critical thinkers.

**Figure 7.8**

## Activity

### Giving praise

1 Consider how you give praise to children. Do you give children praise that focuses on their efforts and on the processes they used in their learning or on the end result – the product?

2 Discuss with colleagues how they praise children to focus on the learning rather than the outcome.

3 Observe some children playing and note down the learning processes they are using. Can you see how they made use of what they know, have a go, try out something new, concentration and keep on trying?

4 Do they show a sense of achievement?

5 Would you be able to give them feedback on the processes you saw them use?

## Motivation: Encouraging active learning

It is when children are self-motivated – motivated from within – that effective learning really kicks in. This is active learning that engages the brain and the body, and results in children challenging themselves and persisting. How parents and practitioners support it is vital, so we need to be doing this in the best way possible.

### Tune in to the children

- Tune in to the children by talking to parents/carers about their child's interests and concerns and observing the children.
- When you have tuned in well you can extend the child's interests and learning by adding different resources linked to their interests, for example, information books or stories that may extend ideas or provide information. Remember that the most effective learning takes place for young children when the activity and exploration is chosen by the child.

### Know when to join in

- Before you join in with children in their self-chosen activities and play, stand back for long enough to work out what they are focusing on. Then join in as a fellow investigator who is interested in what they are interested in, or as a play partner, so that the children remain in control. Sometimes you will need to stand back for longer or not get involved at all at this point.

### Partnership with parents

- Talk regularly with parents about what children are doing at home, sharing with them what the child is doing in your setting.
- Work out plans together as to how best to support the children to celebrate the processes of learning and help children to become independent, confident and motivated: in other words, active learners. This is important for all children but particularly important where a child has additional needs.

### Provide a stimulating environment

- Provide interesting and stimulating things to do, which will both extend children's current interests and help them find new ones.
- Sometimes setting up the provision in a different way will prompt and extend interests.
- At other times, allowing children to return to the things they have been exploring and concentrating on is more important, for example, keeping children's constructions at the end of the session so they can return to them the next day – or for several days until their involvement has moved on.

### Encourage children to make their own choices and decisions

- Encourage the children to make their own choices, as well as decisions on how they may want to do things. There will be many children to cater for, and as they make decisions and choices they are learning about other people and their choices, too.
- Helping children to negotiate with each other and to play and explore together, especially from the age of 2 years onwards, is an important part of the role of the practitioner.

## Being involved and concentrating

### Flexibility

- Be flexible in your planning so that plans can be adjusted to ensure children can extend their explorations and investigations and become or continue to be deeply involved.
- Reflect on your routines: do they help or get in the way of sustained involvement?

### Develop involvement levels

- Note whether babies and children are becoming deeply involved. If some children are not, what can be done to help?
- Think about the learning environment: is it supporting children's interests and providing new ones? Is it inclusive of every child's interests and learning needs?
- Think about how practitioners work with the children: does this encourage involvement or cut across it, perhaps by requiring children to come and do other activities when they are busy concentrating.
- How do adults talk with the children? Questions need to be used carefully. When questions are used, are they open-ended enough?
- Think about time: do children have enough time in their self-chosen activities. Do adult-led activities give time and space for children to explore and follow their own line of thinking?

## Keeping on trying and enjoying what they set out to do

### Enable all children to participate

- Observe the children to ensure they are all able to participate fully in learning and that they are encouraged to persist in their learning.
- Make sure you have the level of challenge right for the children. If things are too easy or not stimulating enough, children will become bored and disinterested, and when this happens they either switch off or find it difficult to behave appropriately. If things are too difficult they will be put off trying.

## Provide the right amount of help

■ Make sure that children's learning has the right amount of help; not by doing things for them, but by giving them just enough support. Sometimes this will mean breaking things down into smaller steps.

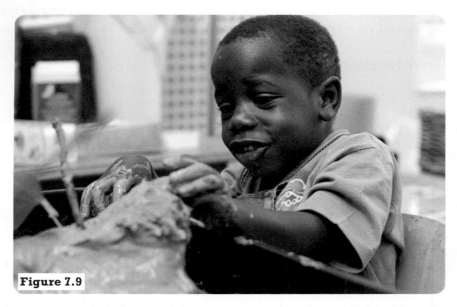

**Figure 7.9**

## Encourage persistence

■ Avoid imposing incentives and rewards as these tend to demotivate children in the long term. They may have short-term and immediate gains, but children will all too easily come to rely on these and only be motivated to do hard things if it is linked to a reward.

■ Talking with children about their learning and the learning processes they are going through or using will help to keep them motivated.

## Take care when giving praise

■ Praise children's efforts and be specific about praising the processes of learning. This will support them to keep trying and enjoying what they set out to do, at the same time as giving them the vocabulary to reflect on their own learning.

■ When you praise the children, use words such as exploring, investigating, figuring it out, trying again, concentrating, listening to other children's ideas, cooperating. Soon they will be using these words themselves.

## Chapter summary

This chapter will have helped you:

➤ understand what active learning means and the three aspects highlighted in the EYFS

➤ recognise when children are engaged in active learning and what deep-level learning looks like

➤ think about the kind of child-initiated and adult-led activities to provide for children to ensure they are learning.

## Further reading and references

Dweck, C.S. (2007) *Mindset: The New Psychology of Success*, Ballantine Books, New York

Evangelou, M., Sylva, K., Kyriacou, M., Wild, M. and Glenny, G. (2009) 'Early Years Learning and Development: Literature Review', DCSF Research Report RR176. Available to download from: www.education.gov.uk/publications/RSG/publicationDetail/Page1/DCSF-RR176

Laevers, F. (2000) 'Forward to basics! Deep-level-learning and the Experiential Approach', *Early Years*, Vol. 20, No. 2

Laevers, F. and Lulo, H. (eds.) (2003) *Involvement of Children and Teacher Style: Insights from an International Study on Experiential Education*, Leuven University Press

National Strategies/DCSF (2007) 'Confident, Capable and Creative: Supporting Boys' Achievements', National Strategies/Department for Children, Schools and Families, London, available to download from: www.foundationyears.org.uk

Stewart, N. (2011) *How Children Learn: The Characteristics of Effective Learning*, Early Education (The British Association for Early Childhood), London

# Chapter 8

# Creating and thinking critically

## In this chapter we will be looking at:

➤ what creating and thinking critically means and why this is important in children's learning

➤ some observations of children developing their creativity and critical thinking skills

➤ the views of experts who have helped develop our thinking about how best to support learning

➤ what effective practice looks like.

## Introduction

Creating and thinking critically is the third of the three characteristics of effective learning highlighted in the EYFS 2012. Although we briefly discussed it in Chapter 4, this chapter tells you more about it.

Being with children when they are creating and thinking critically, and helping them to develop their thinking skills, can be one of the most exciting aspects of working with young children.

## The EYFS tells us:

*"When children have opportunities to play with ideas in different situations and with a variety of resources, they discover connections and come to new and better understandings and ways of doing things. Adult support in this process enhances their ability to think critically and ask questions."*

(EYFS card 4.3)

What could be more exciting in our work with young children than this!

Here is Isobel, aged 4 years, being given an opportunity to think about her own learning. The staff in this school share the significant achievement books (learning diaries) with all the children regularly, and also with their parents. Isobel was looking at her significant achievement book, which is full of observations and photos of her busily involved in many activities, most of which she has chosen to do. Isobel is asked: "Looking through your book, which parts do you like the best and feel most proud of?"

"I made this model with the blocks and then I knocked it down. I wanted to do it again, but I couldn't remember how to do it. Sandra showed me the photograph."

Turning the page, Isobel said, "This is my favourite page." She looks at a photograph of herself with a paper mask on her face. "I made the mask all by myself. I did all the drawing on it. It's just got one eye-hole." Moving on to another page, she said, "I really like this too. Look, I made a mermaid. I cut out her tail and decorated it."

Sharing the children's achievement books or learning diaries with them in this way gives them a really useful opportunity to look back and ponder on their own learning. It helps them to think about their own learning and development and the next steps. As Nancy Kline says, "Everything we do depends for its quality on the thinking we do first" (Kline, 1998).

## The EYFS characteristic of learning, Creating and thinking critically, tells us:

Creating and thinking critically are ways that children make sense of their experiences. As the Tickell Review put it:

*"As they engage in activities they actively think about the meaning of what they encounter and over time begin to develop more awareness of their own thinking. Awareness of oneself as a thinker and learner is a key aspect of success in learning."*

(Tickell Review, 2011)

As with the other characteristics of learning, reception class teachers are required to complete information for Year 1 teachers on aspects of creativity and critical thinking. They are closely linked to the other characteristics of learning, play and exploration, and active learning.

## What is this characteristic of learning about?

Creativity and critical thinking are two different concepts that are closely related. *Creativity* in this sense is not about creative development or the arts, but is to do with the way we think and feel: it involves seeing things in new ways, making new connections, using imagination to develop thinking and generating new ideas. This does not mean ideas that no one has thought of before, but new ideas and new ways of thinking for *this particular child*. It is an important aspect of being human; it is not about being talented. *Thinking critically* is about developing the kind of reflective thinking that helps us to organise our thoughts and think things through. It involves reflecting on and developing awareness of one's own learning, and learning how to learn, just as Isobel, at the beginning of this chapter, is being helped to do.

The EYFS 2012 has highlighted three components or aspects to creating and thinking critically:
1 **Having their own ideas**
2 **Making links**
3 **Choosing ways to do things and finding new ways.**

Each of these aspects will be looked at in turn to help explain how children develop their creativity and critical thinking, and how adults can facilitate their development.

# 1. Having their own ideas

Generating ideas involves using creativity and new ways of thinking. As the Tickell Review puts it: "Being inventive allows children to find new problems as they seek challenge and to explore ways of solving these" (Tickell, 2011). Being inventive is part of creativity. When we think of creativity we also think about the enjoyment of the process. This may be personal, but we often want to share this with others.

## Creating and creativity

Our creativity helps us to figure things out by using our imagination and thinking of possibilities, and being flexible and open to new ways of seeing and doing things. Creativity is very evident in the way that babies and young children approach exploration and play. Their curiosity about everything around them means that they are exploring constantly. As babies become mobile and develop into toddlers we see them using any object within reach as something to explore. As they grow, imagination becomes more visible and audible.

Sometimes young children create their ideas on their own, but often they want to be with other children in a collaborative venture, even though it is more complex when other children's ideas have to be accommodated. It is easy to see when observing children involved in cooperative play or carrying out an activity together how their creativity and imagination helps them to:

■ plan what they want to do and how to do it
■ find interesting problems to solve
■ try to solve them.

These are vital elements of creativity that children need in their daily lives.

## Communication and creativity go hand in hand

An important aspect of creativity is being able to communicate our thoughts and ideas to others. This requires us to think through what we are doing – by being able to share it with someone else. We often hear young children, particularly 2- to 5-year olds, talking to themselves as if giving a running commentary, perhaps describing to themselves what they are doing or narrating the storyline of their play. Often they are planning out loud what to do next. Sometimes you will even hear this self-talk or private speech in the midst of playing with others, so some of the talk is to their peers and some to themselves. If we listen in we can tell so much about their thinking. As children get older, this private speech really does become private, internalised into inner speech. Even as adults we often catch ourselves thinking aloud in this way too. So, talking to ourselves and talking to others helps us to organise our thoughts and think about new possibilities. However, there are many ways of communicating, and although language is important it is not the only way. Loris Malaguzzi, the founder of the Reggio Emilia approach, which you may have heard of, calls this the Hundred Languages of Children.

## What we can do to help?

Children need time, space and encouragement for their creativity and creative thinking to blossom, and the early years setting is the ideal place for it. This has implications for how practitioners interact with the children, particularly helping them to think through what they are doing. Getting involved in play alongside the children, encouraging their imaginations and possibility thinking will help, showing that we enjoy this too. "When children are encouraged to think about 'what might be' instead of 'what is' the sophistication of their thinking is often revealed" (National Strategies/DCSF, 2010).

# 2. Making links

This really does bring together critical thinking and creativity. It starts as young babies organise the information they receive from using all their senses and movement. Gradually, children develop greater control of the thinking process so that they are able to make connections more consciously and deliberately. Much of our thinking appears to happen in an automatic way, but we are constantly planning what to do next and thinking of possible ways to do it. For all of us – children and adults alike – being able to reflect on how we came up with particular ideas or new ways of seeing something is important.

## Using language to support thinking

As children become more verbal, language becomes a very important tool for thinking. Although the 2012 EYFS does not specifically highlight language for thinking, this aspect of language is vital to children's learning. It is through *expressing* thoughts that we often come to understand things in greater depth or in a new way. Explaining things is a key aspect of thinking critically.

How we interact with children as we involve ourselves as partners in their explorations and play makes all the difference in helping them to develop awareness of their own thinking and learning. In What the experts say, later in this chapter, you will read about some of the research on sustained shared thinking and the ways in which practitioners interact to extend children's learning. As Marion Dowling says, practitioners "are able to enter the child's world, recognise his/her interests, dilemmas and concerns and have a conversation which encourages further thinking" (Dowling, 2005).

We can encourage children to ask BIG questions like Louis, age 4 years, who asked me: "How did the world get made?" Helping him to express his thoughts and working collaboratively by getting involved in further investigations supported his thinking. "Through listening to young children, respecting their thoughts and feelings, sharing the joys of their discoveries and understanding their motivations, practitioners can create environments where each child's unique strengths, interests and fascinations can unfold" (National Strategies/DCSF, 2010).

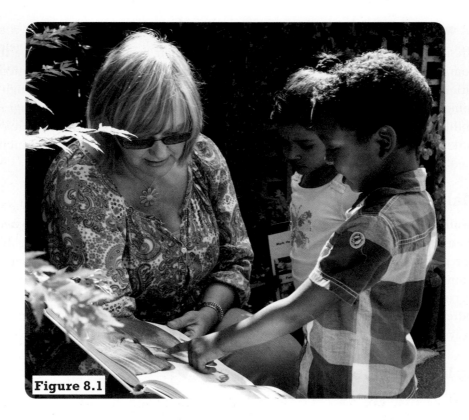

**Figure 8.1**

It may be one child who sparks off a new idea or investigation, but involving a small group of children who may have similar interests is likely to snowball into more interesting questions to investigate. Trips out are a brilliant source of first-hand experience to support any investigation. Information books and searches on the internet, as well as targeted imaginative stories, can fire the imagination to provoke children to ask questions and develop ideas.

## 3. Choosing ways to do things and finding new ways

This final aspect of creating and thinking critically involves "making choices and decisions about how to approach a task, planning and monitoring what to do, and being able to change strategies" (Tickell, 2011). Research shows that when children are involved in self-chosen activities they are more likely to want to find the right strategy than if an activity is adult-directed. Encouraging children to investigate and experiment gives them the experience they need to begin to organise their thoughts and figure out how to proceed. Successful learners do not see mistakes as insurmountable problems, but as challenges to try again. Having a variety of strategies to hand is important.

### Thinking about thinking and thinking about learning

Some of the most important skills children need for the future are the ones that involve them in reflecting on their learning. The support provided for Isobel and her peers to talk about their achievements at the beginning of the chapter is one way of doing this. Recent research has shown that when children are asked *how* they solved a problem, they learned more than when they were just given positive feedback on solving the problem (Evangelou *et al.*, 2009). Conversations about the learning processes children are using are important in helping them to develop awareness of their own learning, using open-ended questions such as "How did you manage to do that?" or "What helped you do that?" Research shows that we do not hold these types of conversations nearly often enough with children in the early years or in school. At first, children who are not familiar with this way of working may need us to help them become aware of the skills and knowledge they have applied, through talking with them about what we have seen them do. Sharing something about your own learning is also helpful: "I really have to think about that", or "I am not sure. I wonder how to do that? I will need to find out more."

Pat Gura and Lorraine Hall point to the need to introduce much more talk with children about their learning: "If children's awareness of their own thinking is to develop, they need to hear adults using words like

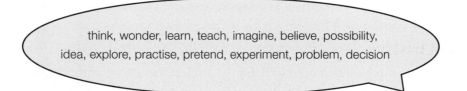

think, wonder, learn, teach, imagine, believe, possibility, idea, explore, practise, pretend, experiment, problem, decision

… as they play and work with children. Adults who think, imagine, plan and remember aloud also help demonstrate the processes involved" (Gura and Hall, 2000).

## Activity

How often are the words listed in the quote above used in your day-to-day interactions with the children? Try to make time for infor\mal discussions with children about their play and the activities they spend most time at. Talk to them about how they are learning and thinking.

### Helping babies and toddlers to develop creativity and critical thinking

Throughout this chapter there have been suggestions and ideas as to what we might do to support older children (from 3 years upwards). But what about babies and toddlers? Giving babies and toddlers plenty of safe and interesting things to explore and time to do this helps to support creativity and critical thinking skills. Elinor Goldschmied developed the idea of treasure baskets for sitting babies; and for mobile babies and young toddlers she developed what is called heuristic play (heuristic means discovery; see below). These provide opportunities for under-2s to explore in a deeper way, and as they do so they are:

- engaged in active learning
- choosing or rejecting objects
- matching, sorting and categorising
- developing awareness of the properties of the objects
- organising their thoughts.

## Treasure baskets

Treasure baskets can be introduced to babies at around the age of 6 months, when they can sit up but are not yet crawling. A basket made of natural fibres is provided *once* it has been checked to make sure there are no sharp edges and that it is stable for a baby to pull themselves up on it. In the basket is placed a collection of safe objects made of natural materials, with different textures, shapes and weights to offer different sensory experiences.

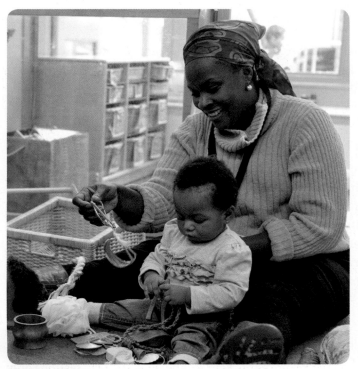

**Figure 8.2** Treasure basket

Careful selection of objects and materials is needed for variety and safety. The basket may contain things like a fir cone, a pebble or two (big enough to be safe, but not too heavy), a few shells of different shapes, a soft ball, a pompom or bath lily, a soft brush such as a body brush (check that hairs are secure in the brush), a set of keys, a sponge, a loofah, a cork, a lemon and a wooden spoon or small rolling pin. Often a piece of soft, see-through fabric is included too.

Ensure that the babies are in a quiet and calm space, with the key person/adult quietly observing, showing interest. A new object can be offered from time to time that has not yet been noticed, but it is important not to interrupt the baby's explorations and flow. When interest wanes it is time to move on to something else. While they are exploring the babies will be:

- selecting objects of interest
- exploring using all their senses
- grasping things in different ways
- seeing what happens if they drop, bang or wave an object.

Physical experiences come together with sensory experiences to develop thinking.

### Heuristic play

A heuristic play session is a planned session for children in their second year of life, usually taking place once a week. This is a quiet time for the children to explore real objects and materials uninterrupted. It needs *pre-planning*, considering how, when, where and how often to offer it. A quiet, warm, comfortable floor space, large enough for the resources and the children, is needed. Access to toys and other equipment should be limited to allow children to concentrate on the heuristic play, by covering other equipment with drapes.

The children are provided with large quantities of at least ten collections of different types of objects, made, as far as possible, of natural materials.

## Heuristic play materials

Cardboard tubes, wooden cotton reels (if available), jar lids, short lengths (half a metre or so) of metal chains, corks, woollen pompoms , curtain rings, wooden dolly pegs (make sure they are not spring pegs and that the wood is smooth and not splintery), ping-pong balls and more. Ideally there should be between 40 and 60 items of each type.

Each type of object is sorted and carefully stored, for example, in drawstring bags and in a cupboard, to use just for the heuristic play. Receptacles such as deep metal biscuit tins or catering tin cans (making sure edges are not sharp) are also needed for the children to put the objects into or to stack, roll or explore, as they wish.

The practitioners prepare the room, setting out the resources in separate piles.

During the session practitioners keep as quiet as possible, staying seated near the children, showing interest in what they are doing and only intervening to show a child a different set of resources if a conflict arises. There is no set length of time and the session should continue until interest wanes, perhaps up to 30 minutes. Tidying up is very much part of the session, so that the children help you sort and collect the items into the right bags. It needs to be unhurried, using simple instructions to the children.

Although treasure baskets are increasingly used in settings, heuristic play is less common, but equally important. This is often because of the time and planning involved in finding the right materials in the quantities needed without explicitly hunting for them. However, craft shops and craft materials websites can be very useful sources. Chains can usually be bought in a DIY/hardware store and cut to the length you want. As the resources are kept for the heuristic play sessions only, they keep well, although some, such as the cardboard tubes, need replacing regularly.

# Looking at children:
## What do we see?

### Renee, age 1 year

The heuristic play is set up ready for the older babies and toddlers. This nursery uses heuristic play for babies from 10 months to toddlers of about 18–20 months.

Renee becomes very interested in the chains, dropping then into tins and pulling them out again (see Figure 8.3). Her concentration is deep and she is completely absorbed in exploring the features of the different chains for the next 15 minutes or so. In Figure 8.4 you can see how, having explored the other chains, Renee is pulling one to see what happens.

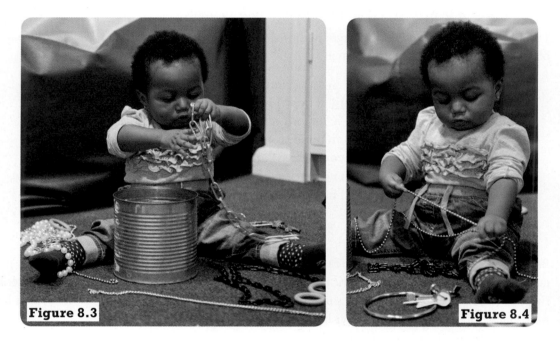

Figure 8.3                Figure 8.4

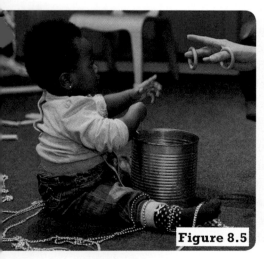

Figure 8.5

After a few minutes, she looks up and her key person wonders if she is interested in other objects. She shows her some wooden curtain rings and metal bangles. She takes them and explores them, continuing her deep involvement until the session ends.

### What have we found out?

The room is quiet and contemplative, although some of the babies are quietly babbling to themselves. There is enough space and resources to enable Renee to continue her involvement uninterrupted by the others. This has helped her to stay deeply involved in her explorations with the chains. She feels the links, drops one into a tin and takes it out again and repeats this several times. She explores the difference in feel and weight of the chains – you can see her thinking.

## Malachy and Advan, age 4 years

Dinosaurs have been a popular imaginative play resource with a group of boys lately, so the dinosaurs are always easily accessible. Malachy had recently been taken to the Natural History museum by his family to see the dinosaurs. Today dinosaurs were available in the water feature in the garden and several boys chose to play with them. After a while, some children moved on to other things, but Malachy and Advan stayed.

Then Malachy said, "You know, I saw a film on telly about the dinosaurs and a meteor hit the earth and they all died." The practitioner, Judy, replied: "Why do you think that happened, Malachy? Why did they die?"

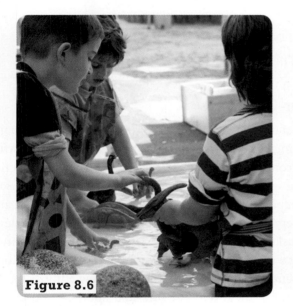

**Figure 8.6**

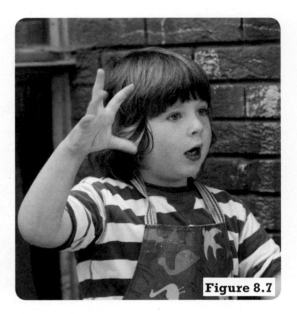

**Figure 8.7**

Malachy: "There was lots of dust and it got very dark and stopped all the trees growing and the trees died and there was nothing for them to eat."
Judy: "Did they all eat plants then?"
Malachy: "They like to eat leaves."
Judy: "Are they vegetarians then?"
Malachy: "Yes."
Advan: "No, dinosaurs eat meat."

Some discussion about meat eaters and vegetarians followed, then Judy said: "Ah, perhaps the meat eaters died because there were no plant eaters left to eat." The conversation continued for a while, with Malachy, Advan and Judy agreeing among other things that dinosaurs lived millions of years before humans.

### What did we find out?

Malachy wanted to share his new knowledge and a discussion ensued, sustained by the interest of the practitioner. Both children already know a lot about dinosaurs: about what they ate, for example. The new fascination was why they died out and how dust could have brought this about. The practitioner was important in sustaining the conversation, joining in as an equal partner and thinking of possibilities with the children. She showed real interest in what they were saying. Later, sharing this learning story with Malachy's mother, she mentioned his interest in the meteorite and why living things might die. In the coming weeks the staff will plan to follow up the children's interests, investigating the ideas raised further.

## What the experts say
### Improving practice and shared thinking

### Improving practice with under-3s

Elinor Goldschmied was a nursery teacher and psychiatric social worker who has had a major influence on practitioners working with young children in the UK and around the world. After retirement and well into her nineties, she continued to support the development of effective practice with under-3s in day care settings. She was one of the authors of the 2002 book *Key Persons in the Nursery*, discussed in Chapter 2 and published when she was 92 (Elfer, Goldschmied and Selleck, 2002). Goldschmied was not only very influential in developing the key person system, she also developed the practice of treasure baskets and heuristic play. The ideas were first written about in the book *People Under Three* that she wrote with Sonia Jackson in 1994. A second edition was published in 2005, with Goldschmied remaining as a consultant to the new edition. As the authors say in the preface to the second edition, they were not sure that another edition was needed: "The unanimous view of our advisers was that although the early years scene had indeed been transformed the book still occupied a unique place in the sparse literature on day care for under threes." Even though things have moved on since 2005, it remains a very valuable book. She also produced videos on treasure baskets and heuristic play that are now available on DVD.

### Sustained shared thinking

The project *Researching Effective Pedagogy in the Early Years* (REPEY) (Siraj-Blatchford *et al.*, 2002) is part of the Effective Provision of Preschool Provision (EPPE) project. Both projects have been discussed in What the experts say sections in other chapters. The REPEY research looked in detail at some of the data from the EPPE project to examine why some settings resulted in significantly better outcomes for children. One of the most important findings was about the nature of the interactions between staff and children, and the ways in which children's thinking and ideas were supported. They noticed that:

*"…in the excellent and good settings, the balance of who initiated the activities, staff or child, was very equal, revealing that the pedagogy of these effective settings encourages children to initiate activities as often as the staff."*

(Siraj-Blatchford *et al.*, 2002)

They define the word pedagogy not only as how the staff interact with the children, but in terms of the context they provide too, including the learning environment, relationships with parents and routines of the day. One of the most important outcomes of this finding has been the expectation in the UK that in the early years there will be a balance of adult-led and child-initiated activities.

The most significant finding was that best outcomes for children were linked to:

*"… adult–child interactions that involve 'sustained shared thinking' and open-ended questioning to extend children's thinking".*

(Siraj-Blatchford et al., 2002)

Sustained shared thinking is the term that the research uses for the best quality interactions that are likely to lead to learning. It is "… an episode in which two or more individuals 'work together' in an intellectual way to solve a problem, clarify a concept, evaluate activities, extend a narrative, etc. Both parties must contribute to the thinking and it must develop and extend …" (Siraj-Blatchford *et al.*, 2002). It can only happen when practitioners have a good awareness about the child's interests and understanding. Although it does not happen very often, when it does, it makes a difference to children's achievements. It happens most when the practitioner extends interactions that the child has initiated. "Freely chosen play activities often provided the best opportunities for adults to extend children's thinking" (Siraj-Blatchford *et al.*, 2002).

## Effective practice:
## What do we need to do?

### Setting up a learning environment

Setting up your learning environment, inside and outside, as a place that encourages creativity and thinking makes a big difference to children's learning. This means unrushed but stimulating, with interesting things to discover, explore and provoke children to ponder on, and, most important, *time* and *encouragement* to do so. The role of the adult is to be a facilitator to thinking, supporting children to explore, experiment and investigate and come up with their own questions.

### Creating a thinking environment

Nancy Kline's research has shown the importance of the thinking environment for adults to improve their thinking skills. Her research shows that we rarely provide the types of environment for people to think for themselves or for thinking and creativity to flourish.

*"The best conditions for thinking are not tense. They are gentle. They are quiet. They are unrushed. They are stimulating but not competitive. They are encouraging. They are … both rigorous and nimble"*

(Kline, 1998)

Creating a thinking environment starts by listening attentively to each other. Kline believes we are not very good at this. Think of the number of times in a conversation that someone else talks over you or finishes your sentence for you. This is because you have sparked off their own thinking and they are no longer listening to you! When this happens, they tend to take over the conversation and your thinking is blocked. This happens with adults talking to adults, but it happens even more when we talk to children. And as well as doing this with young children, we have a tendency to ask them lots of questions, most only requiring one-word answers. We do not do this on purpose, but we do do it. None of this helps children to use their imaginations, think about possibilities and have new ideas or figure things out for themselves. So effective practice means we need to think hard about how to improve our thinking environments.

## Having their own ideas

### Partnership with parents/carers

- Talk with parents about what children are showing interest in at home, so that you can follow their fascinations. Talk about what you are doing and how you are encouraging children to have their own ideas and choose their own ways of doing things.
- Talk to parents about the ideas children are exploring and showing interest in in your setting, so that they can follow up these ideas in the home as well.

### Encouraging exploration

- Plan plenty of opportunities for exploration, allowing children time to explore, investigate and discover – in groups or alone. Choices for what to explore need to be relevant to the children, so knowing what the children are showing interest in is the starting point. Sometimes it is best to stand back and let the children explore uninterrupted; at other times, getting involved as a fellow investigator or explorer is important. Asking open-ended questions might prompt children into trying out new ways of doing things.
- Provide plenty of opportunities for babies and toddlers to explore safe but interesting objects and toys, appropriate to the child's age. Develop treasure baskets and heuristic play sessions.

Remember, materials and resources need to be well organised and thoughtfully presented if they are to help develop children's imagination, creativity and thinking skills. Finally, tidying up is important and part of the heuristic play.

### Encouraging imagination and creativity

- Support children's interests, so that they can develop over time.
- Do not change the provision too often, especially when children are showing particular interest. Let the children develop it with you over time, by asking them for their ideas – for example, in developing a role-play area or needing to find space for a new resource.
- Provide opportunities for children to express their own ideas.

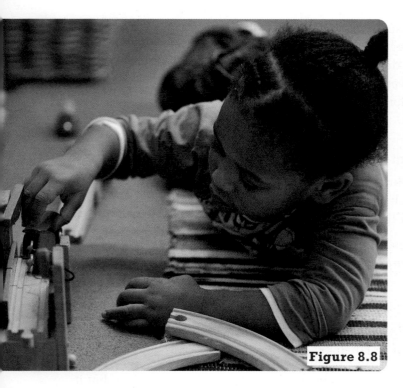

**Figure 8.8**

## Making links

### Problem solving

■ Respect and encourage children's own ideas, by showing interest and encouraging them to follow these up. Imagination can be fired by reading imaginative stories, especially ones that show the main characters discussing possibilities, being inventive and resourceful.

■ Support children in finding problems to solve through their play, through activities and through discussion. For example, suggest they help to design a water feature in the garden or a new climbing frame, or something really practical, such as how to keep the coat rack tidy! The children can make a book with your help about the investigation or experience, through photos of the process and the children telling how they approached the task. Points to note:
  – Make sure that the group is small enough to involve all the children in the discussion.
  – Make use of information books, stories and the internet.
  – Be an attentive listener and take on board the children's ideas.
  – Show genuine interest in what the children have to say.
  – Ask the children to think in advance about how they might go about their investigation.
  – Find interesting ideas and topics to think about and investigate.
  – Ask children for their ideas of what to investigate and encourage them to ask questions.
  – Ask open questions and encourage thinking about possibilities: What if?
  – Ensure all children can be involved by giving children with additional needs support to join in.
  – Share your own thinking with the children so that they see you wondering, speculating or offering an alternative point of view.

### Activity

Next time a problem arises in your learning environment, such as needing a space for a new piece of furniture, or stopping the wash basins from flooding, pose the issue to a small group of children (older 3- and 4-year-olds). Ask them to think of solutions and write down their ideas for all to see. Then try out some of their ideas, discussing with them which idea to try first and how to go about it. (Use the points described in the section Creating a thinking environment to help you.)

## Choosing ways to do things and finding new ways

### Supporting children to reflect on their own thinking and learning

■ Have discussions about thinking and talk to children informally about thinking as you work with them, using the language of thinking and learning, as described earlier in the chapter.
■ Talk to them about different ways of doing things and ask them for their ideas.

### Talking to children about their own learning and sharing records

■ Talk to children about what they have been doing and help them reflect on how they did things.
■ Share their learning diaries with them and then involve them in planning what to do next.

## Activity

Next time you want to change the role play or an area of provision, ask the children what it should be and how to set it up. Then set it up with the children, using their ideas. It is best to always have a home corner, so this would be in addition to the home corner.

## Chapter summary

This chapter will have helped you:
➤ to understand what this characteristic of learning, creating and thinking critically is all about
➤ to recognise the importance of encouraging exploration and investigations to children's learning
➤ to think about how to involve children in reflecting on their own learning.

## Further reading and references

Dowling, M. (2005) *Supporting Young Children's Sustained Shared Thinking: An Exploration* (training materials and DVD), Early Education (The British Association for Early Childhood), London

Dowling, M. (2008) *Exploring Young Children's Thinking Through their Self-Chosen Activities* (training materials and DVD), Early Education (The British Association for Early Childhood), London

Evangelou, M., Sylva, K., Kyriacou, M., Wild, M. and Glenny, G. (2009) 'Early Years Learning and Development: Literature Review', DCSF Research Report RR176. Available to download from: www.education.gov.uk/publications/RSG/publicationDetail/Page1/DCSF-RR176

Gura, P. and Hall, L. (2000) 'Self-assessment' in *Early Years Educator*, June, Mark Allen Publishing

Goldschmied, E. and Jackson, S. (2005) *People Under Three: Young Children in Day Care*, Routledge, Abingdon

Kline, N. (1998) *Time to Think: Listening to Ignite the Human Mind*. London: Cassell Illustrated

National Advisory Committee on Creative and Cultural Education (1999) 'All Our Futures: Creativity, Culture and Education', Report to the Secretary of State for Education and Employment and the Secretary of State for Culture, Media and Sport

National Strategies/DCSF (2010), 'Finding and Exploring Children's Fascinations', National Strategies/Department for Children, Schools and Families, London, available for download from: www.foundationyears.org.uk

Siraj-Blatchford, I., Sylva, K., Muttock, S., Gilden, R. and Bell, D. (2002) *Researching Effective Pedagogy in the Early Years* (REPEY), Research Report 356, Department for Education and Skills, London

Stewart, N. (2011) *How Children Learn: The Characteristics of Effective Learning*, Early Education (The British Association for Early Childhood), London

### Useful websites

Treasure baskets and heuristic play: http://coreexperiences.wikia.com/wiki/Treasure_Basket_and_Heuristic_Play

*Infants at Work* DVD (Elinor Goldschmied) and *Heuristic Play with Objects* DVD (Anita Hughes and Elinor Goldshmied), available from: www.communityinsight.co.uk

Elinor Goldschmied obituary: www.guardian.co.uk/society/2009/jun/12/obituary-elinor-goldschmied

# Section 3: Learning and Development Part 1: The prime areas of learning

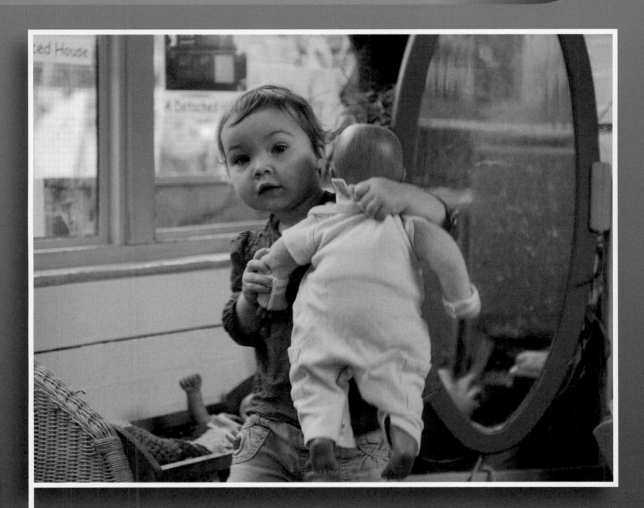

The revised EYFS has designated three areas of learning as the prime areas of learning, because of their importance to child development. The prime areas of learning are:

➤ Personal, social and emotional development (Chapter 9)
➤ Communication and language (Chapter 10)
➤ Physical development (Chapter 11).

As the Tickell Review stated in 2011:

"It is widely agreed by researchers and practitioners that personal, social and emotional development, physical development and communication and language are closely linked to one another and central to all other areas of learning and development".

This section examines these prime areas of learning.

# Chapter 9

# Personal, social and emotional development

## In this chapter we will be looking at:

➤ how children's personal, social and emotional skills develop right through the EYFS age range and how play supports this

➤ observations of children as they develop their personal, social and emotional skills

➤ research by experts in the field

➤ effective practice with a case study showing how one setting has been supporting a child with special educational needs.

## Introduction

Enza has just had her first birthday. She has recently started in nursery, attending for two full days per week. She has bonded well with her key person and parts well from her mother, as well as showing delight when her mother returns. She confidently explores the different areas of the large, well-resourced room and particularly likes to explore the basket of musical instruments. Today she moves from the musical instruments to the water tray, pulling herself up to a standing position and splashing her hand in the water, laughing as she does so. She happily plays alongside the other children here, watching what they are doing.

The under-3s area in this setting is open-plan for much of the day and all the children – the babies, toddlers and young children (some of whom are just 3 years) – use the room together. Enza has settled in well and is very much at ease playing alongside some babies and toddlers of her own age as well as some children who are older. She has adjusted well to the new environment, helped by the care her key person has taken in making a relationship with her and her mother. Her self-confidence is high and she is already making new relationships beyond her immediate family. Children's personal, social and emotional development is always a priority here. We can see that Enza feels secure, welcomed, valued and a part of the nursery community.

## The EYFS prime area of learning, Personal, social and emotional development, tells us:

*"Personal, social and emotional development involves helping children to develop a positive sense of themselves, and others; to form positive relationships and develop respect for others; to develop social skills and learn how to manage feelings; to understand appropriate behaviour in groups; and to have confidence in their own abilities."*

(EYFS Statutory Framework, 2012)

Personal, social and emotional development (PSED) is a prime area of learning. It permeates every aspect of the EYFS because developing confidence and developing relationships with others underpins all other learning. Although there is a broad pattern of development in PSED, every child's development is unique and individual, formed by their own earliest experiences, the relationships that others have formed with them and whether or not the environment provided for them supports their learning and development.

## What is this prime area of learning about?

Our personal, social and emotional development shapes how we respond to every situation we encounter in life. Babies are social beings, and from the very moment of birth a baby is highly sensitive to the responses she or he receives. Social and emotional development is a fundamental aspect of human development. It does not stop when children are 3 or 5 or any age – we continue to develop this throughout our lives as we build new relationships and encounter new experiences.

Research on child development has increasingly emphasised how social and emotional development, together with communication and language, provide the foundation of children's ability to function successfully in the world when they are older. At the same time as young children are developing their personal, social and emotional skills, they are also learning about everything else. And it is what adults do to support children's personal, social and emotional development in the earliest years that has the most significant impact on their future learning and their lives. So we need to start with strong, positive relationships with parents, help children build friendships and ensure a consistent approach to managing behaviour. Getting this support right is vital.

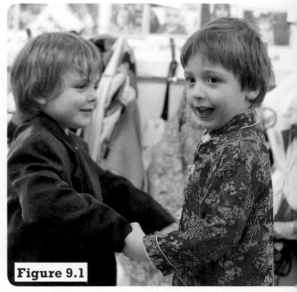

**Figure 9.1**

We talk about *personal*, *social* and *emotional* development as one area of learning, but the three words really cover three different but closely interlinked themes:

- *Personal development* refers to the way we develop awareness and understanding of ourselves as individuals, with our own character and abilities. Successful personal development means that we have a positive sense of self and a positive attitude to ourselves.
- *Social development* is all about developing positive relationships with others and seeing ourselves in relation to other people. Successful social development means we get along with others and feel connected to them.
- *Emotional development* is about how we develop understanding of our own feelings, learn how to express them and manage them effectively. It includes understanding the feelings of others and develop empathy.

**The 2012 EYFS highlights three aspects of PSED. These are:**

1 **Self-confidence and self-awareness**
2 **Managing feelings and behaviour**
3 **Making relationships.**

Self-confidence and self-awareness are related to personal development; Managing feelings and behaviour is a major part of emotional development; and Making relationships and understanding others is social development.

## 1. Developing self-confidence and self-awareness

To support the development of their self-confidence and self-awareness, children need:

- supportive and close relationships with their key person and other practitioners in the setting
- an enjoyable and inclusive experience in the setting, free from stress
- to know that they are valued, respected and cared about.

Babies are highly sensitive to other people's responses to them and much of their learning about themselves, other people and the world around them stems from this. The responses they receive from their main carers affect how they manage their feelings, develop relationships and whether or not they develop self-confidence. When a baby's smile is responded to positively by the adult or crying results in a soothing cuddle, feeding or changing, then they begin to develop self-confidence and awareness that they can influence and rely on others.

We pass our feelings on to children very easily. If we are feeling confident and positive then a child is much more likely to be so too. New parents may be very anxious about doing things right for their young baby or toddler and the anxiety may easily spread to the baby. Practitioners can help to reduce the anxiety by supporting parents, answering their questions and finding additional professional help where this is needed.

Between the ages of 6 months and 1 year, babies are developing a close attachment to those most familiar to them and become increasingly wary of other people. If they are starting to attend a setting at this time – or at a later stage – separation from their main carers needs careful handling. Babies and young children may find separating from their main carer relatively easy or quite difficult. Here the role of the key person in empathising and developing a strong relationship to support the child is vital. A child's self-confidence requires consistent and supportive relationships and frequent conversations between the key person and parents to ensure that the child feels happy, safe and well cared for. You can find out more about attachment and the key person role in Chapter 2.

## Learning from others

From 6 months onwards babies are also beginning to understand other people's responses to new things, in order to find out how they should respond. They are developing self-awareness, but also awareness of others. They look for signs of approval or disapproval in facial expressions and body language and listen out for particular tones of voice. So, for example, if the main carer shows delight or, alternatively, is upset or anxious, then the baby is most likely to show the same emotion.

Juliet Neil-Hall, a specialist in behaviour and early years, lists ten emotional needs that all humans have. These are the need for:

| | | | | |
|---|---|---|---|---|
| Attention | Acceptance | Appreciation | Encouragement | Affection |
| Respect | Support | Comfort | Approval | Security. |

These are useful to consider in developing supportive relationships with children that will enable them to flourish and grow confident, considerate and emotionally strong (Neil-Hall, 2007).

## Activity

1 Discuss the words relating to the ten emotional needs shown above with colleagues in your setting. You could play this as a game by writing each word at the top of a piece of paper and passing it round a circle at a meeting.

2 Each person has to write an example of what they do to ensure they provide this for the children, then fold it over and pass it on.

3 At the end there will be a long list of examples that could be used in a display for parents. A similar activity could be done at a workshop for parents.

## Developing independence

As babies become more mobile they want to try more and more out for themselves, as we saw with Enza splashing in the water tray. By the age of 2 years the development of their physical skills will have made them much more independent and they will be very interested in exploring everything, but they will still need a great deal of adult support to do things for themselves. The support needs to be the right amount, not taking over, nor leaving them to be frustrated, but allowing them to try. Their developing ability to use words to express their needs helps them to tell others what they want.

By the age of 3 years, children making independent choices about what they want to do and play with becomes easier, as their communication and language development means they are more able to ask for what they want. Feeling confident to try new experiences depends not only on supportive relationships with adults, but to an extent on their own personality. An anxious or very shy child will need support. A child with a fixed mindset (see Chapter 7, What the experts say) will need support to become more open. Separating from parents/main carers may continue to be difficult for some children who are less confident, so continuing support from the key person is always necessary.

## Attending more than one setting

Some children may have multiple carers in any one day. For example, they start the day at home, then go to a childminder, who takes them to the early years setting, and are then collected by grandparents before going home. For each part of the day, there may be different expectations about what they are and are not allowed to do. Other children may attend one setting for part of the week and another for the rest. It is important to keep in close contact with parents in these circumstances to ensure the child is not finding all these changes difficult.

## Managing feelings and behaviour

Managing feelings and behaviour is all about emotional development, learning to understand and express feelings and understand and empathise with others. To support toddlers and young children in managing their own feelings and behaviour we need to:

- be aware of the messages our own behaviour might be giving to children
- help children to express their feelings, understand the feelings of others and know what is acceptable behaviour
- ensure routines flow with the children's needs rather than for the convenience of the staff
- be aware that sometimes in play with others, children negotiate very well with each other to iron out differences, but sometimes they need our support
- communicate clearly to children when we want them to do something specific.

When it comes to managing feelings and learning about acceptable behaviour, the only model young children have to learn from is the adults and other children around them. We all want children to become caring, considerate and kind. But they learn from everything we do – both what we want them to learn and what we do not want them to learn. It is worth checking: how aware are we of what our own behaviour looks, feels and sounds like to others?

Watching children in role play, playing at being the adult mummy or daddy or the practitioner reading a story at group time, can be quite revealing when we hear a child using a bossy tone or telling children off. This play is very important to children as they are putting themselves into what they see as the adult role. They are mimicking our behaviour, or how they *interpret* our behaviour. We may think we are not bossy, but children are so attuned to our tone and body language that they may interpret our behaviour in this way. Children learn all about how to communicate from our non-verbal communication – our facial expressions and body language – long before they are able to understand words or talk themselves.

## Learning about behaviour

When emotional development is progressing well, we are able to express our feelings appropriately and empathise with other people. Young children need to find out what our responses are and the best way for them is to test. We may have high expectations of behaviour and often take it for granted that young children know how to control their feelings and behave in acceptable ways. A consistent approach to managing behaviour across the setting is important, ensuring everyone works in a similar way.

Kay Mathieson writes that practitioners need to think of their role as "one of a companion in a journey of joint discovery" (2005) for the child. Children do not learn by being told to be nice to others and to behave well – they learn by trying things out for themselves. Sometimes this can be quite testing for the adults around, requiring us to be calm and clear about where the boundaries are and how far we are willing to be flexible. Regular discussions with parents are also important to develop strategies together as to how to support the children's development.

## Dealing with clashes

As babies grow into toddlers and then 2-year-olds, they want – and need – to do things for themselves. From time to time they are bound to clash with others, for example, if there is something they want that another child is playing with. In this situation, some children will need help to become more assertive, while others may need help to express their feelings in more acceptable ways and understand the feelings of others. The best support we can give them is to help them communicate their feelings effectively and appropriately in words. We all have strong emotions at times, at both extremes: excitement and delight on the one hand, and anger and upset on the other.

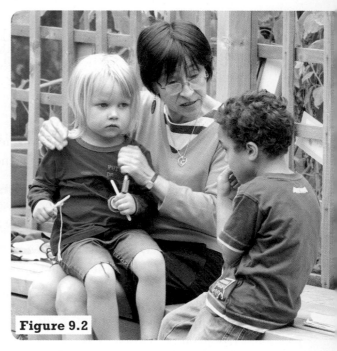

**Figure 9.2**

## Rules and rule-making

With children of 4 years and older, holding regular discussions about friendships and involving them in making the rules for positive behaviour gives children the opportunity to reflect on what it means to be part of a happy community. Persona Doll stories can provide a useful tool for such discussions.

### Routines to support children

Do the routines of your setting support the children to manage their feelings and behaviour? The environment and routines can help, but sometimes they are the cause of some of the problems children may have. Certain times of day, such as group time, tidy-up time or meal times, can be particularly stressful for some children, especially when they are required to stop their play or the chosen activities. We need to consider whether we stop the flow of their play too frequently.

## Making relationships

From the beginning babies are social beings, but attending an early years setting can be the first time that the baby or young child is expected to form relationships beyond close family. To support children practitioners need to:

- help them develop relationships with others
- provide them with the vocabulary needed to help them join others in play
- get involved in play alongside the children, not taking over
- provide activities that require a pair or a small group of children to work together.

### Different types of play

Babies love to be in the company of others they know well and need the attention of the adults they are attached to. They also show a lot of interest in other babies and young children. Between the ages of 2 and 3 years, children become really interested in making relationships with other children, wanting to play with them. At first this may be playing alongside others, but soon, and with sensitive adult support, this will develop into cooperative play. Some children will need more support than others to develop strong relationships with other children. This is partly to do with personality, but also with their experiences of relationships with other children at home.

Play provides the best context for young children to make relationships. There are different kinds of play, from playing alone, which is often called *solitary play*, to playing alongside others, which we call *parallel play* to *cooperative play*.

In parallel play children are playing next to or near each other, and although they may be doing similar things they are not interacting. Any type of play may be either quiet or exuberant and boisterous. As children grow older they begin to play together much more, often making very definite choices about who they want to play with. You will see this most in role play and imaginative play, both inside and in the outdoor area. By the time a child is 4 or 5 years, cooperative play with friends can be sustained for a considerable length of time.

Children play in different ways at different times, usually as suits the occasion. But it must be remembered that young children cannot be expected to cooperate and be involved in cooperative play and games for too long. Just like adults, they need their own space where they can choose what to do without being expected to be part of a group. Most importantly, adults being on hand to give support where and when it is needed is vital to supporting children's development in forming relationships successfully.

# Looking at children:
## What do we see?

### Tanuj, age 2 years 4 months

In this observation we see Tanuj in his first few weeks in the under-3s provision in a Children's Centre where he attends three days a week.

Soapy water has been put out in bowls, with sponges and scrubbing brushes for the children to wash the wheel toys. The children are dressed in waterproof suits. Tanuj begins by exploring the bubbles in the bowl with his hands, then watches two others washing the trikes and joins in, delighted. He then runs around with a brush and tries scrubbing the tree, then the wall, then back to the trikes. "Clean now," he says to the others and "Bike wet." Then he joins the two others washing the caterpillar tunnel.

### What have we found out?

Tanuj is beginning to make friends and the observation shows how play provides the best context for this. In the Centre that Tanuj attends, the practitioners write their observations in the form of learning stories, written as a story *to* the child. These are then shared with the child and the parents. Stella, the practitioner who made this observation, analysed what she had observed: "Tanuj, you seemed to enjoy washing the trikes, exploring the bubbles and the different sponges and brushes. You were very involved all of the time. I noticed you telling your friends about what you were doing as you played alongside them."

### What next?

Stella has noticed Tanuj's interest in making relationships and realises that this is important for him, so she writes, "We will plan for you to take part in similar activities with a small group of children to encourage and support you in making friends." She also lists several other activities and experiences that will be provided to encourage him to explore.

### Samira, age 2 years 8 months

Samira is a few months older and has been in the nursery a lot longer than Tanuj and knows many of the children well. She uses role play and imagination to practise and develop her understanding of the social and emotional world. As with other 2- to 5-year-olds, this is her way of exploring the world of feelings and relationships. Samira was playing with soft toys in the home corner. She took the telephone and phoned the doctor, telling the doctor that her dog's leg was broken. She took a pencil and pretended to give the dog an injection with the pencil. She phoned the doctor again: "I'm feeling better, but my dog isn't," she said. "It's his leg – and his tummy now! Oh dear, he has been sick on my trousers." She then put the dog to bed and read it a story. She covered it in a blanket and gently rocked the dog in the bed. She told another child playing nearby all about the dog's condition. Then she went into the garden and began to ask children if they were well, offering them some medicine and injections.

### What have we found out?

In this observation, Samira shows a sophisticated array of knowledge about caring for the sick dog and looking after others. This is role play, but it seems deadly serious as she takes on the caring mother role. This type of play is a powerful tool for many children to get into the adult's shoes and shows how much they pick up from observing adults around them.

## What the experts say
## Importance of positive adult–child relationships

Sue Gerhardt is a British psychotherapist. In 2004 she published an important book for professionals working in the early years as well as parents, called *Why Love Matters: How Affection Shapes a Baby's Brain*. Just how important others are in a child's development is evident in Sue Gerhardt's work. In the book she explains some very complex neuroscience about the development of the baby's brain and the effect of the type of care the baby receives in shaping the brain. As a result of the response the baby receives from the moment of birth onwards, the pathways of the brain begin to be set. These establish how well we are likely to be able to cope with what life throws at us, not only as babies and young children, but also as adults. "Good early relationships build up the right chemical balance and emotional balance to deal with stress" (Gerhardt, 2004). How we cope with learning and other aspects of life are also affected.

Gerhardt points out that being emotionally available to the baby is key. As she puts it: "the mystery tonic that enables babies to flourish as soon as they get it, is responsiveness... not too much (which would swamp the baby causing stress) and not too little (which would result in stress through neglect) but just the right amount."

## Two-year-olds' testing behaviours

Parents are often concerned by the testing behaviour of their 2-year-olds.

Alison Gopnik and her colleagues Andrew Meltzoff and Patricia Kuhl are professors in child development in the USA. They have carried out extensive research into early childhood development, and in their book *How Babies Think* (2001) they write about all aspects of early development. Their chapter on social and emotional development, "What children learn about other people", provides an accessible synopsis of research into how babies and young children learn social skills and appropriate behaviour. For example, by 9 months babies have already learned to tell the difference between other people's expressions of happiness and sadness. By 18 months they are usually able to understand that their own likes and dislikes and those of other people may not be the same.

The chapter is very helpful in explaining why 2-year-olds behave as they do and are often so contrary in their behaviour – as they call it, the terrible twos. They point out that 2-year-olds are actually *deliberately* perverse: it is an important strategy for learning. "What makes the terrible twos so terrible is not that the babies do things you don't want them to – one year olds are plenty good at that – but that they do things *because* you don't want them to" (Gopnik *et al.*, 2001). They have a powerful need to know how others will react, so they test it out. The authors make a comparison between 2-year-olds and adult scientists testing a theory. The theory they are testing is the differences between their own desires and those of others. The authors also point out how, at the same time all of this is going on, 2-year-olds are also developing empathy for others and can be very caring – just as Samira and Tanuj are in their play.

The book helps us to see that we need to be patient and calm and make our feelings explicit with 2-year-olds, giving them the words for what we think and feel and helping them to understand our reactions when they test us.

## Effective practice:
## What do we need to do?

Building positive relationships with all parents is the starting point to effective practice. Once children have settled in well it is all too easy to take personal, social and emotional development for granted. Sometimes, parents and practitioners just expect that children will automatically get along with each other and know how to behave. But effective practice means we consciously plan for children's personal, social and emotional development; we do not leave it to chance. Remember, everything you provide has an impact on the children in one way or another!

### Ensure consistency

- Ensure there is a consistent approach by all staff to managing children's behaviour and helping children to form positive relationships with others.
- Try to be aware of the messages your own and your colleagues' behaviour might be giving to children. Does it model the kind of behaviour you want children to show, to become caring, considerate and kind?

## Self-confidence and self-awareness

- Ensure that *all* children know that they are valued and cared about. Give children focused praise for their achievements and for good behaviour, being specific about what they are being praised for.
- Observe the children to make sure they are having an enjoyable, fun and relaxed experience in your setting.
- Support children to develop confidence to try out new things. This might mean being a learner alongside the child, showing them that you are trying it out too. Talk about your thoughts with them: "I haven't tried this before but I think I would like to give it a go..."
- Make your own feelings explicit. Sometimes share your dilemmas and ask children to help you to solve problems. Telling children about things you find hard can make children more confident as their opinions are being valued.

### Activity

Provide some enjoyable turn-taking games that help children (from age 3 onwards) to take turns and share. Make sure that children needing additional support can join in with others who are more experienced at sharing and taking turns, so that the latter can act as role models. Let the children take it in turns to be the caller or game leader, while you are there to provide support.

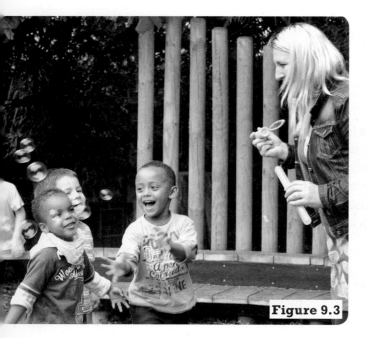

**Figure 9.3**

## Managing feelings and behaviour

- Use the vocabulary children need to express their feelings with them, by talking about your own feelings as well as what you think they might be feeling. Specific planned activities and small group discussions with children about their feelings are very helpful, but make sure they are appropriate to the child's developmental level.
- Ensure routine times, such as group times, cause the least disruption to the flow of the day and that they support the children's needs rather than being convenient for the staff.
- If a child does something that is not acceptable, such as deliberately upsetting another child or adult, ensure the "victim" is comforted and be clear with the child exactly what was not acceptable. Make sure they understand that they are still loved and it was the behaviour that was not acceptable, not the child themself.
- Help children to play with others by giving them the support they need, such as ensuring that they have the words they need to negotiate with others. Don't step in too quickly. Watch and listen first, as children can often sort out their own differences.

- Assist children who need additional support in managing their feelings and behaviour. Observe children who you feel need additional support to find out exactly what triggers unacceptable behaviour. It may be that the child is finding a particular time of day difficult, or particular kinds of play. Once you and others in your setting are clear about the trigger, take appropriate action to support the child.
- Pitch what you say at the right level for the child, to ensure they understand you.
- Ensure every member of staff knows the behaviour management policy and that it is regularly discussed and reviewed by the staff team and shared with parents.

## Activity

### Routines of the day

1 How often do children have to stop what they are doing to tidy up for a group session during the day? What times of day do these take place? Can you explain what the educational purpose is of each of them? Do all children appear to gain from these experiences?

2 Group times – why and how are children grouped? How many times a day? Do some children often seem unsettled or bored? How could you do things differently? If some children are finding it difficult, what can be done to help them? For example, sessions could be shorter, the group could be smaller to accommodate different children's needs better, at a different time of day or there could be fewer group sessions.

## Making relationships

- If you are concerned that a child is finding it difficult to make relationships, observe the child to see how they approach other children so that plans can be made to support them further.
- Help children to form relationships with others by being available to support. If you see a child on the edge of play or observing others playing, talk to them about what they are watching and ask them if they want to join in. You can then show the child how to join in. This may start by you both playing alongside the other children doing something

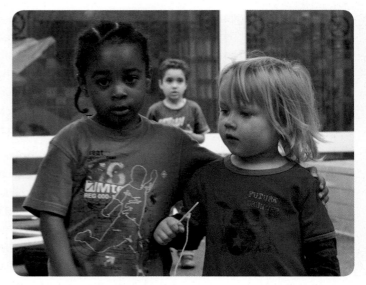

**Figure 9.4** Children learn to be caring and to look after each other

similar to their play, then gradually getting more involved in joining the group, providing the child with the vocabulary needed to ask if he or she can join in.

- Answer parents' concerns about children building friendships and getting along with others and discuss your setting's approach to managing behaviour. If possible, hold meetings and workshops for parents about how children's behaviour and friendships develop.
- Provide experiences that require two or a small group of children to work together, such as wheel toys for two children and other outdoor equipment. Tidy-up time can help – for example, putting the large blocks away together, or two children needed to carry a piece of equipment safely. Sometimes set up specific activities. You can choose children who have shown some interest in each other because they may have similar play interests or ways of approaching things.

## Case study: St Anne's Nursery School and Children' Centre: Support for Johann

The Nursery School and Children's Centre caters for all the children who attend. Staff plan carefully to meet their individual needs and support them to become active participants in the vibrant nursery learning community. Johann, who started at the school at 3 years old, has additional needs. The very close relationship between the school and his parents has been the key factor in ensuring that his needs are met, frequently reviewing his progress together to ensure he is learning to his full potential. Partnership with outside agencies has also ensured that any need for additional specialist support is met. The support he has received in the school and at home has developed his confidence and enabled him to progress in all areas of development. His mother said: "The support from the school has been amazing and very informative."

Through talking with his parents and through their observations the school staff know well Johann's particular strengths and interests, for example, his interest in and enjoyment of stories and books and his love of painting. They also have a firm understanding of the areas in which he needs additional support and plan together to ensure the most appropriate support. Johann receives one-to-one support from a Senior Nursery Officer with experience of working with children with additional needs. A fundamental aspect of the support has been to ensure he is fully included in the nursery day, learning with his peers within the rich and stimulating learning opportunities created for all the children. Johann's mother feels that the close relationship he has built with the Senior Nursery Officer and other staff has been very important to him.

Johann has been supported in his understanding of the routines and patterns of the day, through regular reminders and direct teaching of particular skills. His language and communication development has been supported to ensure he understands what is said, modelling the vocabulary he needs to talk about what interests him and to express his feelings. By 4 years 5 months Johann was able to communicate verbally very clearly to others about some of the routines of the day. In this observation from his learning diary he is able to explain turn taking to a staff member (a sand timer is used from time to time to help the children take turns at the computer): "When the sand is finished it's M's turn." When it did, he gave the mouse to M, saying: "I give it to M. Look, the sand is finished, it's her turn."

## Chapter summary

This chapter will have helped you:

➤ understand more about the EYFS and personal, social and emotional development
➤ find out about what some experts are telling us about children's development in PSED and the role adults play in supporting this
➤ reflect on your own practice and the practice in your setting.

## Further reading and references

Gerhardt, S. (2004) *Why Love Matters: How Affection Shapes the Baby's Brain*, Routledge, London

Gopnik, A., Meltzoff, A. and Kuhl, K.P. (2001) *How Babies Think*, Orion Publishing Group, London

National Strategies/DCSF (2008) 'Social and Emotional Aspects of Development', National Strategies/Department for Children, Schools and Families, London

Neil-Hall, J. (2007) 'Attachment: Supporting Young Children's Emotional Wellbeing', *Early Years Update*, July

Mathieson, K. (2005) *Social Skills in the Early Years: Supporting Social and Behavioural Learning*, Paul Chapman Publishing, London

Paley, V.G. (1993) *You Can't Say You Can't Play*, Harvard University Press

# Chapter 10

# Communication and language development

## In this chapter we will be looking at:

➤ how children acquire language and develop communication skills

➤ children at different stages in their development in communication and language, including one child learning English as an additional language

➤ some research by experts in the field about how best to support children's communication and language development

➤ what is effective practice, with some tips, activities and a case study showing how one setting has been supporting a child to become a skilful communicator.

## Introduction

Communication and language development begins at birth. Like all babies, at birth Ellie was already familiar with the sound of her mother's voice. She looked intently at the face of the person holding her and from a very short time after birth she could imitate some of their facial expressions, such as pursing her lips, opening her mouth or sticking her tongue out. Her mother and father and others around give her intense, loving and caring attention, talking to her and attending to every sign she makes of discomfort or contentment all her waking hours. By 6 weeks old she gives beaming smiles when making eye contact with someone holding her close and smiling at her – she expects a response or turns away. At 7 weeks, when her mother talks with her and she is feeling comfortable and relaxed, she gazes into her mother's face, holding her gaze for a few minutes, already taking turns in making sounds in a conversational way. It is difficult to know who starts this sequence of sounds – does Ellie start and the adult copies or is it the other way round? Whichever it is, already a conversational-type of behaviour is becoming well established.

Communication and language are essential tools for life: we cannot function independently without them. They incorporate all the skills we use to communicate with others around us through words, gesture, facial expression and body language, as well as the skills we use in listening to and understanding others. From birth rapid development in communication and language takes place. By the time children are 4 or 5 years most can expertly negotiate with others, express their own thoughts and ideas, give instructions or report back on what they have been doing – and a lot more! How has this been possible? It has not happened alone: even though we may not be very aware of what we as adults have done, our interactions have been crucial from the very moment of birth.

## The prime area of learning, Communication and language development, tells us:

"Communication and language development involves giving children opportunities to experience a rich language environment; to develop their confidence and skills in expressing themselves; and to speak and listen in a range of situations."

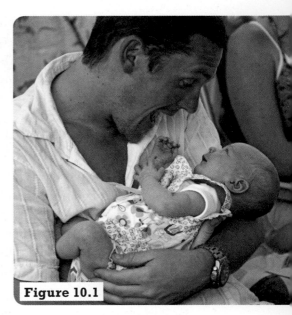

**Figure 10.1**

(EYFS Statutory Framework, 2012)

As communication and language development is a fundamental aspect of child development, the revised EYFS has designated it as a prime area of learning.

## What is this prime area of learning about?

The EYFS divides communication and language into three aspects as these are the essential elements needed to become a skilful communicator:

1 Listening and attention
2 Understanding
3 Speaking.

Differentiating between the aspects in this way helps us to pay close attention to each and think about what we need to do to provide the necessary support. We need to remember, however, that communicating is essentially a *social* activity – we do it to communicate something to someone else – so *how* we use language is also very important.

■ *Listening and paying attention* to what is being communicated or said by others is essential for communication to work.

■ *Understanding* focuses on whether the meaning of what others have said has been fully understood. We often call this receptive language. It is not always easy to know whether a child has understood what has been said, without observing them closely. We may unwittingly make assumptions that children have understood the words, when they may have guessed what was said from the context or gestures.

■ *Speaking* is often called expressive language. A child's development in expressive language is much easier to assess as we can hear what they say and how they say it.

Although the EYFS divides communication and language development into these three aspects, babies and young children are acquiring and developing all three aspects simultaneously, and they do this through interacting with those around them. As children are learning to communicate effectively, they are also learning a great deal about everything else too. So, to put it simply, as children learn to communicate they are also communicating to learn!

## Why not communication, language and literacy?

Communication and language became an area of learning in its own right in the EYFS in 2012. Until then the EYFS combined communication and language with literacy. However, putting literacy with communication and language often meant that we were not paying enough attention to supporting the development of communication and language development. In 2006 I CAN, a charity that supports children with speech, language and communication difficulties, published a paper which noted that more than 50 per cent of children in England were entering school with some kind of communication difficulty, which, with the right support, would be solved.

With this in mind, in 2008, a government-funded programme, Every Child a Talker, was developed, with the aim of ensuring that practitioners in early years settings and parents were better informed about children's language development and how to support it. The emphasis on improving our support for children's communication and language skills still continues.

As a core element of child development, communication and language is a prime area. Literacy, on the other hand, depends on children knowing and being able to use a body of knowledge. It is therefore a specific area of learning. Although this helps us understand and plan for both areas of learning better, it does not mean that the two areas of learning are any less closely linked. It is not a case of one then the other. The wonderful opportunities provided by the world of books for babies and older children remain as important as ever for learning about language, as well as developing early literacy skills. From board books and bath books for babies, to the exciting and absorbing story and information books for 3- to 6-year-olds, books provide a rich resource for looking at, listening to, talking about and enjoying. When read aloud they provide a wealth of opportunities to hear the rhythms and flow of meaningful language, building anticipation as the page is turned, developing children's imagination, thinking, knowledge and understanding through language. In addition, we cannot learn to read and write without being competent and skilful communicators.

For the older end of the EYFS age range, continuing support in communication and language is essential – it continues throughout education until adulthood, as we refine our skills in communicating in different ways and for different audiences and increase our vocabulary.

## Acquiring and developing language and communication skills

Acquiring and developing language and communication skills usually follows a similar pattern. However, some children need additional support, and the earlier this is given the better. This is why it is so important to look at all three aspects of communication development, so that the right support can be given.

## Learning to talk: The first few months

Eye contact is important from the very beginning: babies gaze into the faces of carers holding them close and from as early as 20 minutes after birth, babies are already able to imitate some mouth movements of the carer. Their communication is deliberate, with cries showing the need for attention, and gurgles and smiles showing satisfaction. For much of the time it is the baby who initiates the communication and the carer who responds.

How we respond is important. Even though there is no understanding of the words yet, the baby is making sense of the tone, sounds and rhythms of her or his language. Taking turns to communicate develops very early. As babies begin to coo with deliberate, contented sounds (by about 9 weeks old), most adults automatically respond in the gaps the baby leaves and vice versa. As with Ellie, it is often hard to know whether this dance-like conversation is initiated by the adult or the baby!

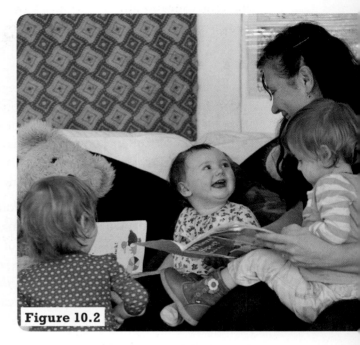

**Figure 10.2**

From about 6 to 7 months, babbling begins – repeating and experimenting with a wide range of sounds, tones, volume and pitch. Babbling is important: this is when babies are practising all they will need later when they begin to form words. Communication and language experts such as speech therapists hope that babbling will have started by 11 months, so look out for it if you are working with this age group. By 12 months infants usually respond to their own name by turning to look at whoever spoke. Understanding words, particularly names of people and objects develops rapidly now, as can be seen by the infants' responses – such as pointing, looking at or touching the object in response to a simple "Where's the/your …?" question.

## First words

Normal language acquisition follows a similar pattern across the world. Although there is no strict timetable, with plenty of warm and supportive attention from caring adults through conversation-like interactions, smiles, giggles and having fun, by the time most infants are between 10 and 15 months the first recognisable words appear. We help by giving our attention, simplifying our speech, emphasising particular words with an exaggerated or sing-song voice, playfully repeating words and sounds. Alongside this are fun turn-taking games, such as peekaboo, with plenty of repetition, gesture and facial expressions. Once words start to appear vocabulary is acquired rapidly, particularly naming people, objects and animals. At this stage one word may stand for many similar things, such as "wow-wow" or "goggy" for any four-legged animal.

Some parents introduce 'baby signing' to their babies between the ages of about 9 to 18 months, to help them communicate their wants and needs – just as Emma's parents did in Chapter 5. This is easy for babies to pick up, but words must be used too, as this is just an *aid* to communication.

## Putting words together

By the age of 2 years children should be beginning to put two to three words together and there is almost an explosion of learning new words. At first this will be in a form of truncated speech where only the most significant words that ensure others understand are put together. In terms of listening and attention, although there is a tendency for the child to be deeply absorbed in one task at a time, when the child's attention is called they are generally able to focus on what they are being asked to do. They frequently show us how much more they can understand than say.

As speech develops further and more words are put together it becomes clear how quickly children have picked up the rules of grammar, such as the past tense. You will often hear children of 3 and 4 years saying, "I goed" instead of "I went", having understood the rule about adding -ed to make something past tense, but not yet knowing all our irregular verbs. At the same time as children manage to grasp the rules of our grammar and become increasingly proficient at understanding longer sentences said to them, they are able to convey more complex points and speak more complex sentences themselves.

## Talking to learn

Communication and language, like social relationships, is at the heart of being human. It is also a main vehicle for learning about everything else. As Gordon Wells, who we will hear more about in What the experts say, put it, just like adults:

*"Children talk to achieve other ends: to share their interests in the world around them, to obtain things they want, to get others to help them, to participate in the activities of the grown up world, to learn how to do things and why things are as they are, or just remain in touch"*

(Wells, 1986)

They also ask questions to find out what we think and how things work. The most important aspect of the language environment we create for children is providing the time and encouragement for them to want to communicate with us and with their peers.

### Signing and alternative communication systems

Some children will need additional help to communicate effectively. Signing is the most common form of support, using a programme such as Makaton or Signalong. These are used with speech and provide additional support through making specific signs. Makaton also has picture symbols which can be pointed to. To use either system, you and everyone involved with the child will need training. Some children, such as those who are profoundly deaf, are likely to need an alternative sign *language*, such as British Sign Language.

## Activity

This activity is suitable for those working with children age 2 years and above.

1 How much time do you allow for meaningful informal conversations with the young children in your setting?

2 Does your setting enable children to communicate and use language in all the ways shown in the grid below?

3 Are children who are learning to talk using signing or using an alternative communication system able to communicate in these ways too?

|  | Yes/No |  | Yes/No |
|---|---|---|---|
| Expressing needs, wants and wishes |  | Making comparisons |  |
| Expressing feelings |  | Clarifying thoughts and ideas |  |
| Negotiating with others |  | Reflecting, evaluating |  |
| Explaining |  | Clarifying understanding |  |
| Asking questions, enquiring |  | Developing ideas with another person/ people |  |
| Giving reasons |  | Expressing imagination |  |
| Describing |  | Making predictions |  |
| Reporting information |  | Making suggestions |  |
| Giving instructions |  | Making decisions and plans |  |

## English as an additional language and becoming bilingual

Many settings will have children learning English as an additional language (EAL) and becoming bilingual or even multilingual. Some children are becoming bilingual from birth, others will be in an English-speaking environment for the first time when they arrive in your setting, although they may have been exposed to English through the television and radio at home. Being bilingual or multilingual is a great asset and benefits children's all-round learning, as well as their ability to remain in touch with their family, culture and community. The importance of encouraging parents to continue to ensure their child is fluent in their first language(s) cannot be emphasised enough.

In many ways learning EAL for young children in an environment such as your setting, where they are surrounded by English, is much like learning their first language, but there are some important differences. For children who are beginning to learn English when they come to your setting, they will already have developed in their first language and will be drawing on their experience, knowledge and skills. As with the language, with help, they will be able to understand more at first than they can say, and usually talking begins with one-word, then two-

and three-word sentences. Often young EAL learners go through a silent period, when they are not yet confident to speak in the new language. Do not worry, but do keep on talking to them, making sure you help them understand what you are saying by giving lots of visual clues and encouraging the children to be involved in everything that is going on.

## How does our interaction with children help them to develop?

There are so many things we do as we interact with children, some of which have been explained in this section, but when we are concerned about a child's communication and language development we need to check that we are doing all we can to support them. As Gordon Wells puts it:

*"Talking with young children is very much like playing ball with them. What the adult has to do for the game to be successful is, first, to ensure the child is ready, with arms cupped, to catch the ball. Then the ball must be thrown gently and accurately so that it lands squarely in the child's arms. When it is the child's turn to throw the adult must be prepared to run wherever it goes and bring it back to where the child really intended it to go"*

(Wells, 1987)

# Looking at children:
## What do we see?

### Daisy, age 2 years

At 2 years old, Daisy appears to be particularly interested in the names of any object around her and is developing skilful communication. She listens to what she is told in the course of her everyday experiences and her parents are amazed at how quickly, with very few repeats, she seems to be able to pick up new words, as well as how quickly her sentences have developed. They have noticed that her sentences can be 10 to 12 words long.

As Daisy was playing with a collection of shells at home with family, one family member named a type of shell in her collection as an "mm" shell (as the opening looks like pursed lips). Daisy immediately replied: "That's a cowry. Where's my periwinkle shell?"

Later, Daisy is involved in pretend play with a teddy. She is feeding teddy in a baby chair at the start of this observation, talking to him as she does so:

"I eat my dinner, Mummy, I going straight to bed now… Oh dear, it's upside down now... I need …" (and she creates a long list of things she needs to take with her and teddy to bed).

She then goes off to put teddy to bed:

"You're beautiful …" She starts to read teddy a story: "Let's turn over the pages. Daisy give you that book, Piggle. Now get into bed. Say night, night Daisy Do, Piggle Do. Daisy – thank you. I flying off in my aeroplane now. In your bed now. Daisy got to go to bed with my Piggle. I got to get my book. Daisy got to go to bed. Oh I dropped my stone..."

## What have we found out?

In the observation, Daisy remembers the vocabulary she has learned, demonstrating her listening skills. The second observation also shows how she can reinterpret and reconstruct what an adult says.

In this sequence Daisy is not only talking to the teddy, but also giving a running commentary to him about what she is doing – much like adults do with her. Most of her grammatical constructions are right. Notice how she sometimes uses "my" and "I", and at other times refers to herself as Daisy. This is probably because she is in a transition stage, moving from the earlier stage of always referring to herself as Daisy into the more sophisticated and mature use of "I" and "my".

## Ayoub, age 3 years 5 months

Ayoub speaks Arabic with his family at home. He was at a very early stage in learning English when he first attended part-time in the nursery class about a month before this observation.

Ayoub is sitting at the play dough table. He takes a piece of play dough and says, "Roll it," then picks up a dough cutter and says, "Ginger man." He presses the cutter shape into the dough: "It's big ginger man," and then sings, "Ginger man, Ginger man" over and over. As he continues to press the cutter into the dough he says, "Push, push." He notices a train cutter: "Oh, look a train. Oh, train is going." He breaks the dough into smaller pieces. "Train is going, lots of train, put train there, push push."

## What have we found out?

This observation was recorded by Ayoub's key person, who was present at the activity with him and other children and also took several photos of him. When he saw the photographs he pointed, saying laughingly: "Me, me! Ginger man." Ayoub is relatively new to speaking in English, but is fluent in his first language. The supportive environment in the class and relationships with the adults around have helped him feel confident to use the new language, English.

# What the experts say
## Babies are very capable communicators

Colwyn Trevarthen is Emeritus Professor of Psychology and Psychobiology at Edinburgh University. Through his research he has given us some very significant insights into babies' and young children's development in communication and language over many years. He has also been a great supporter of early years practitioners, being careful to explain his research in ways that we can easily understand. You will find useful videos of him talking about some of his work on the Scottish education department's website (www.ltscotland.org.uk).

Trevarthen's research has shown the sociability and astounding capabilities in the communication of babies and infants. His research has shown the very close coordination of the expressions, gestures and sounds of the baby with those of the mother, developing the same rhythm together. He calls these proto-conversations. One of his particular interests has been in how babies' and infants' sensitivity to the rhythms and gestures of language and communication helps them develop their powers of expression. He has been able to use his research to help parents and those working with young children see how our interactions support babies' and children's abilities to express themselves.

His analysis of adult speech to young children has revealed the importance of the rhythm and tone in developing communication skills. Trevarthen's most recent work is looking at the importance of musicality of language and how movement and rhythm are integral aspects of language, in tune with the melodic patterns of speech.

## Gordon Wells and the Bristol Studies

From 1969 to 1984 an important research project was carried out in Bristol, entitled Language at Home and at School. It has taught us a great deal about young children's language development and the best conditions for it to flourish. Gordon Wells was the Director of the Bristol Studies. This longitudinal study not only followed the communication and language development of a group of children, but in particular the language environments and adult interaction – both at home and at school.

The study initially involved recording 128 young children and their families in their homes at random times, so that no one would know when the tape recorder was on and therefore would not perform to it. The recordings began when some of the children were 15 months old and others were 3 years old and continued for two years – for some children this included recording them at school too. Several books were written on the project by Wells, one of which is *The Meaning Makers*: *Children Learning Language and Using Language to Learn* (1987).

The enormous amount of data has been very useful to us in finding out what are the best ways to support children's language development in the home and at school. Wells is in no doubt about the importance of informal two-way conversations with children, where the child is treated as an equal partner in making meaning. Most of the points he makes are incorporated into what we now know is the best practice in teaching and working with young children. In *The Meaning Makers* he summarises how we can best help children learn to talk in this way: "encourage children to initiate the conversation and make it easy and enjoyable for them to sustain it" (Wells, 1987).

## Effective practice:
### What do we need to do?

### Listening and attention

#### Face to face

- Make sure you are down at the child's level so that you can make eye contact and both of you can see and hear each other well.
- Most important for all children, make sure that you treat anything the child is attempting to communicate as important and worthy of your full attention. This helps to boost their confidence, but also means they will not be frustrated by not being understood.

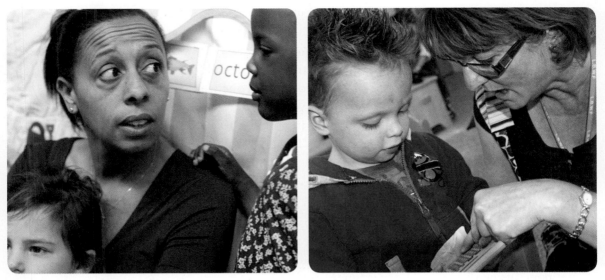

**Figure 10.3**

### Follow the child's lead

- Watch and wait before you talk. Listen intently and pay good attention. Focus on what the child is doing or showing interest in and follow the child's lead! That way you will be on the right track for them to listen and understand you.
- Give the child time to formulate anything they want to say before you start talking.
- Support children who use alternative forms of communication such as signing to initiate the conversation.

### Helping children's attention and listening

- Help to focus the child's attention when you want them to listen to you by saying the child's name first.

## Understanding

### Repeat the child's words back to them

- Repeat the child's work back to him or her and in the process add a little more. This is usually called recasting and is a really useful strategy. When you do this you are doing two things: first you are able to check you interpreted what they said correctly and then you are modelling some new vocabulary or a different way of saying it. For example, if the child says "want bike", you might say – "you want to ride the bike?"
- Keep your vocabulary and the way you say it just a little more advanced than the child's, so you are introducing just enough new things, not swamping them. For babies and toddlers who are not yet saying many words, plenty of repeats of simple phrases is helpful, especially if this is made into a game.
- Do this too when using an alternative communication system for a child who needs additional support.

## Speaking

### Limit your questions

- Research shows us that in early years settings we ask children far too many questions and most often they are closed questions that only need one-word answers.
- Making lots of short comments on what you are doing or see the child doing helps you to limit your questions and then ask them in an open way that encourages children to talk. "Why" and "How" questions work best – "I wonder what/how/why ...?" is a good opener.

### Running commentary

- Comment on what you see the children do in a simple commentary, especially if there is little talk. Do not use too many words, and keep what you say at the right level for the children. You are modelling the words for them. For some younger or less verbal children, your sentences may need to be very short, such as at the dry sand: "pour the sand, pour the sand", or even just "pour, pour", using gesture and body language as well.
- Use signing such as Makaton to help. For more verbally competent children your sentences will be longer and more complex. In this way you can then add an open question too.

### Leave pauses: silence is golden!

- Leave pauses and give children time to think. Many of us hate silences in conversations: it makes us feel uncomfortable and we feel we have to fill the gaps. But for young children it often takes time for them to formulate what they want to say.
- Silences are fine; continue to show you are interested, but do not fill in all the gaps, and give children time to respond.

### Activity

1 Where do children talk most? Check where children seem to do most talking and communicating: how can you develop more spaces for talk?
2 Where are the adults? How often do they get involved too?

### Extending

- Extend what a child says, making sure what you say is at the right level for the child. Most of the points above will help you to extend what the child is saying, and in so doing provide scaffolding for their thinking and language, expanding the conversation.
- Remember, do not talk too much, do not talk for them and leave them plenty of time to talk with you.

## Noise levels

- Think about your setting – how noisy is it?
- What background noise is there that may make it difficult for children to hear?
- Where are the quiet spaces for quiet talking spots?

## Meaningful conversations

- Plan plenty of time for one-to-one conversations or for conversations with children in very small groups. The best conversations are informal and flow easily, as both partners develop their thinking, often from one topic to another or from one angle on a topic to another. This is just the same for children as it is between adults. During this process children are being creative, developing their thinking and ideas as well as expressing their feelings.
- Making sure there is a member of staff who is not timetabled to initiate a planned activity, and whose role it is to get involved in children's self-chosen play as a play partner is essential.

## Have plenty of interesting things to talk about

- Build an element of surprise into what you plan – perhaps a new activity or something set out in a new way.
- Sometimes share something about yourself or your family. This makes the connection for children with what they do at home and can get the conversation flowing.

## Books, stories, songs and rhymes

- Books provide such great opportunities for language – not only by reading them, but also talking about the pictures.
- Having stories told to them is also an important experience for children because it provides a wonderful opportunity to develop children's listening skills and will fire their imagination.
- Start by telling well-known traditional tales. Make the story really active, so children can join in with the actions and a repeating line, such as: "Run, run, as fast as you can, you can't catch me I'm the gingerbread man." Songs and rhymes sung and said are a must – everyday, many times!

## Involving parents

- Find out from parents how they think their child's language development is progressing at home.
- Make sure you talk regularly with parents about their child's language development and what can help. Let them know how your setting is supporting children's language and communication development.

## Activity

Plan a workshop for parents about some aspects of children's communication and language development, with some practical activities, such as introducing new rhymes and songs or talking about books or story props and how to use them. Give plenty of time for the parents to give you examples of what their child does at home.

## Supporting children learning EAL

Children in the early stages of learning English as an additional language need all the things that other children need, but to ensure that they can be fully involved in everything that is going on they also need the following:

- Plenty of visual clues to what we are saying, through our gestures, but also using real objects and photos if we are talking about something that is not present.
- Support to enable the child to relate to the other children if there is no common language between them, by being on hand as a play partner in the group. Explain that the child speaks another language at home and how clever they are to be learning English too.
- Support for the parents in keeping up the child's first language. This not only helps the child to learn English, but helps them socially – as they will be able to communicate with family, friends and the community around them in their first language. It also helps cognitive development.
- No pressure! It is tiring learning a new language. If children are not yet ready to speak in English, continue to involve them in everything that is going on, making sure there is no pressure to speak.

## Case study: Chingford Hall Preschool: Supporting communication and language development

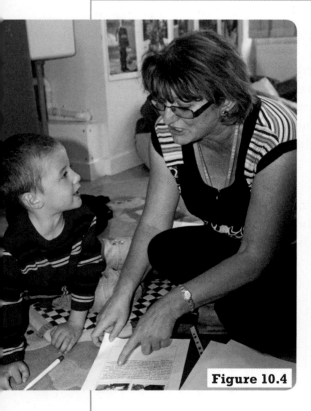

**Figure 10.4**

Chingford Hall Primary School's preschool is part of the Children's Centre and caters for 2-year-olds. Austin started at the preschool part-time at just over the age of 2 years. His key person, Donna, has worked closely with his mother so that they both provide him with the support he needs for his communication and language development. He has also received support from the Speech and Language Therapy Unit. An Individual Education Plan (IEP) has been drawn up by the Speech and Language Therapy Unit and the preschool's SENCo to plan the support for him.

Over his time at the preschool Austin's language development has progressed really well, and he is much more able to understand and express himself now, although he will still continue to receive support. His mother is really pleased with his development and the support he has had at the preschool. Some of the strategies that Donna has used to support him are:

- supporting him in his play, following his interests and keeping what she says to phrases of no more than two or three words, to ensure he can understand and repeat these
- sharing favourite picture books with him regularly and talking about the pictures; he then takes these home to share with his mother

- a daily short group session with Austin and two others, where they sing nursery rhymes with props in a song sack and use the nursery rhyme posters displayed on the wall, share a book or use musical instruments to make contrasting quiet and loud sounds
- an occasional one-to-one session with Austin.

The staff in both the preschool and the school record their observations of the children in the form of 'Learning Stories'. The key person makes an observation and takes photographs when the child is deeply involved in play or an activity. This is written up into an illustrated Learning Story using the photographs. It is then shared with the parents and the child, and is often displayed on the wall too. Austin loves sharing his Learning Stories with Donna and this has been a really good way to help his language development too. You will find the Learning Story in the final chapter.

## Activity

1 Have you had a meaningful conversation with all the children you are responsible for today? This is particularly important if you work in an open-plan setting.

2 At the end of the day, think about your key children: which children did you really spend meaningful quality time with, where you could communicate with each other in a significant, conversation-type exchange?

3 Make a list of those you did not spend much time with and ensure you make time for them the next day. It is best if you do this every day and ask other team members to do the same.

## Chapter summary

This chapter will have helped you:
➤ understand why communication and language have become a prime area of learning
➤ find out more about how children develop communication and language skills
➤ ensure that the way you and your colleagues interact with the children supports their communication and language development.

## Further reading and references

Bercow, J. *et al.* (2008) *The Bercow Report*, Policy Document, Department for Children, Schools and Families, London

Hartshorne, M. (2006) *The Cost to the Nation of Children's Poor Communication*, I CAN Talk Series – Issue 2, I CAN, London

Wells, G. (1987) *The Meaning Makers: Children Learning Language and Using Language to Learn*, Hodder and Stoughton, London

## Useful websites

Colwyn Trevarthen video interviews: www.ltscotland.org.uk/video/p/video_tcm4637499.asp

There are four video interviews here, but also search the Learning and Teaching Scotland site for useful materials on early years (www.ltscotland.org.uk/earlyyears/index.asp).

I CAN: www.ican.org.uk

You will find out more about Makaton at: www.makaton.org.uk; and Signalong at: www.signalong.org.uk

National Literacy Trust: www.literacytrust.org.uk

There are many different sections on the National Literacy Trust website, including one for the early years sector and one for Talk to your Baby.

Talk to your Baby: www.talktoyourbaby.org.uk

This is a really useful site for practitioners and for parents. The Professionals section takes you to the National Literacy Trust, who run Talk to your Baby, but this is a separate site, with video recordings, advice, and so on.

## Chapter 11

# Physical development

## In this chapter we will be looking at:

➤ the pattern of children's physical development and the importance of this to all aspects of learning

➤ children of different ages and different aspects of their physical development

➤ what some experts tell us about how to nurture children's physical development

➤ how we can best support children's development through effective practice.

## Introduction

Two-year-old Daisy is at home with her family. Her aunt has come to stay with her baby – causing great excitement for Daisy. First thing in the morning Daisy runs in to see her aunt, who is sitting on the sofa feeding her baby. A plate of grapes has been placed for Daisy on a low table on the other side of the room. Daisy picks up a grape and walks around the bed on the floor, to the baby and her mother. She looks, chats, eats the grape and returns to the plate again, around the bed but this time walking backwards. This is no easy matter as she has to navigate her route, feeling her way along the edge with her feet and twisting to look behind her. She repeats this little journey several times until all the grapes are gone, each time walking backwards. It has become part of a challenging, self-directed and fun game. Her facial expression shows her delight in her achievement. After her first two trips she only looks behind her occasionally. No one has asked her to move in this way, although the adults around do tell her it is "an interesting way to walk"!

What has motivated Daisy to challenge herself physically in this way and what is she learning from it? We can see that Daisy is very motivated, *wanting* to try out a new skill. She is being playful, willing to have a go and she is certainly concentrating and enjoying achieving her goal (travelling between the fruit and the baby). She has chosen a new way to move, her very own idea, and in the process she is developing her physical skills. At the same time she is:

■ developing her awareness of space

■ finding a new and interesting way to move

■ improving her sense of touch as her feet feel the edge of the bed

■ building her confidence and showing enjoyment.

By the age of 3 years, the physical development of most children has enabled them to learn to walk, run, twist and turn, jump, roll and romp about, use both hands to pick up things, use some tools, pull, push and carry. A great deal of this has been aided by adults who provide the appropriate environment and the physical and emotional support necessary. Physical development includes developing the physical skills that enable children to control their muscles and move in coordinated ways, as well as hand–eye coordination, a sense of balance, and an awareness of one's own body and how to look after it. It is a fundamental aspect of child development. Along with personal, social and emotional development, and communication and language, it is a prime area of learning in the EYFS because it underpins all other learning.

Exploring and experimenting with ways to move, such as Daisy is doing, should be a normal everyday event for babies and young children, but do we encourage children enough to move freely? There is much concern about the increasingly sedentary lives we all lead. Making physical development a prime area of learning in the EYFS 2012 helps us to think more about the importance of physical development to all learning. In the past we have tended to take children's physical development for granted in the early years, unless a highly visible difficulty is noticed. Is there more we could be doing to support children's healthy physical development?

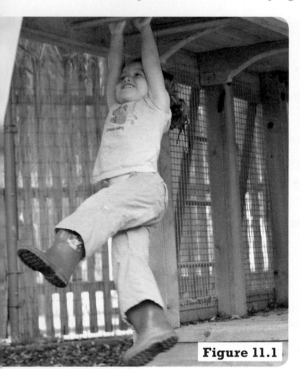

**Figure 11.1**

## The EYFS prime area of learning, Physical development, tells us:

*"Physical development involves providing opportunities for young children to be active and interactive; and to develop their coordination, control, and movement. Children must also be helped to understand the importance of physical activity, and to make healthy choices in relation to food."*

(EYFS Statutory Framework, 2012)

In making physical development a prime area of learning, the Tickell Review stated: "This is a prime area of learning and development because children engage with the world, supporting all their learning, through movement and physical sensations. Through physical play children discover and practise skills of co-ordination, control, manipulation and movement" (Tickell, 2011).

As Penny Greenland, Director of Jabadao, agrees: "It is active involvement and exploration through movement play that enables a child to become a more mature, efficient organiser of sensory information, providing the foundations for all learning" (Greenland, 2006). Physical development is a key area of development examined in the Healthy Child developmental checks made by health visitors. At the 2-year-old health check, the health visitor monitors general development, including movement, growth, speech, social skills and behaviour, hearing and vision. Healthy eating and diet are also discussed with parents.

## What is this prime area of learning about?

Two aspects of physical development are highlighted in the EYFS 2012. These are:
- **Moving and handling**
- **Health and self-care.**

Moving and handling covers those physical skills that enable children to move (gross motor skills) and to control small movements (fine motor skills). Movement involves balance and awareness of the body and body position, as well as actually moving. Fine motor skills enable children to use their hands and fingers (and toes) to handle and manipulate an enormous variety of objects, from large to small, and to use a variety of tools.

Readers familiar with the 2008 EYFS and the Foundation Stage before that will recall that one element of Writing, which came under the area of learning Communication, language and literacy, was about Hand-writing, as this is basically a *physical skill.* In the 2012 EYFS it has been incorporated into physical development.

Health and self-care is about helping children to understand how to be and keep healthy, but it begins by ensuring that we support the children in being healthy through healthy food and common-sense hygiene. Rest and sleep are also very important for development. It is also about developing skills in self-care, eventually managing skills such as dressing and undressing, washing hands and managing the toilet on their own.

### Why is physical development so important?

Experts in child development the world over conclude that young children need to be physically active and moving in order to learn. "Experience gained during physical activity promotes brain development as well as strengthening muscles and the cardio-vascular system" (Tickell, 2011). However, great concern was also expressed about the "sedentary lifestyles at home and in early years settings" (Tickell, 2011), which can interfere with children's physical development, leading to health issues.

The 'Early Years Learning and Development: Literature Review' (Evangelou *et al.*, 2009), undertaken as part of the review of the EYFS 2008, highlighted some key research about a widespread lack of emphasis on physical activity in schools and many early years settings. Over recent years in the UK, outdoor learning and plenty of free play out of doors has increasingly been promoted as a necessity for healthy development and learning. But we still have a long way to go!

## Physical development in babies and young children: What to expect and what to look for

Physical development usually follows a sequence, and as Sally Goddard Blythe notes, "Each stage is important in securing and integrating previously learned skills, and each child progresses at his own rate" (Goddard Blythe, 2011). A useful guide for both the sequence of gross and fine motor development and guidelines for practitioners can be found in *Childcare and Education* (Bruce *et al.*, 2010).

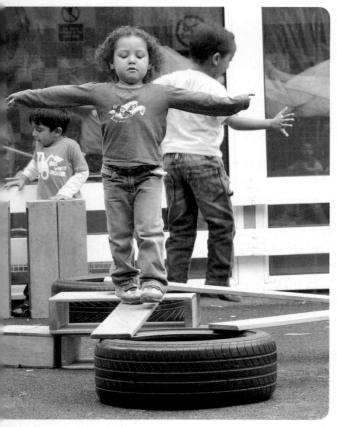

**Figure 11.2** Practising balance in play

## Moving and handling

### Balance and awareness of the body

Every mother is aware of how movement begins early on in the womb. The sense of balance also develops well before birth, but every movement of the mother is cushioned and there is a feeling of weightlessness. Once the baby is born this sense of balance needs to develop in a very new way, to cope with gravity and a very different type of space. Goddard Blythe refers to balance and awareness of where the body is in relation to everything else as two additional "internal" senses. She points out that "it will take a young child many years to use the system efficiently" (Goddard Blythe, 2011).

Balance, awareness of the body and body position are very important. They help the baby to sit upright independently after a few months, and later to crawl, run, hop, jump, climb with confidence and skill, ride a scooter or bicycle or balance on a beam. Goddard Blythe reminds us of another very important point about the development of the sense of balance: "the most advanced level of movement is actually the ability to stay totally still ..." (Goddard Blythe, 2011).

### Gross motor skills

Moving and handling in the EYFS concentrates on movement, coordination and control of large and smaller muscles – from a young baby who at first is able to lie, move arms and legs vigorously and grip with the whole hand, to a baby of 7 to 8 months old who can usually sit up and stand with support, giving the baby a whole new perspective on the world. It is usually not long before moving begins in the form of crawling or bottom shuffling. For most young children, walking independently is likely to be a few months away, but many children begin walking at 9 months, although for others it may be 18 months. Physical skills and development take place in a sequential pattern, helpfully explained by Bruce *et al.* in the following sequence:

- *from simple to more complex* (for example, walking before hopping)
- *from head to toe* (developing control of the head before other parts of the body)

- *from inner to outer* (limbs before fingers and toes)
- *from general to specific* (the example the authors use is showing pleasure, which for a baby is "a massive general response", moving the face and limbs excitedly, but for an older child is more likely to be a broad, beaming smile and words (Bruce *et al.*, 2010).

### Promoting gross motor skill development and balance

The key role for practitioners, as Greenland says, "is to create a learning environment in which children can take the lead in finding activities and games that precisely fulfil their sensory needs both indoors and outdoors" (Greenland, 2006).

### Floor play and tummy time

For babies, being able to play freely on the floor, lying on their backs and on their tummies, is important for developing balance, muscle tone and strength. Once the baby can sit up unaided it is important that they are able to do this freely, to establish balance and muscle strength. It is not only babies who need time on the floor – it is the best place for so much development across the age range.

### Outdoor play

Outdoor play is a statutory requirement in EYFS for good reason. Children need to roll, rock, swing, slide, spin, tilt and purposefully fall for fun. These actions help them to develop balance, and support both gross and fine motor skill development. Obviously, outdoor play is essential to achieve this. Children also need some planned, fun, physical games giving them the opportunity to experience and develop all these skills. Rough and tumble play is important, although often practitioners worry that children will hurt themselves. However,

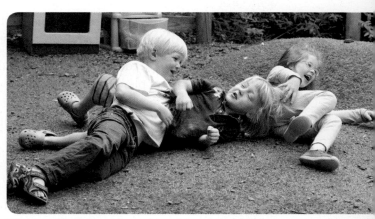

**Figure 11.3** Rough and tumble play whilst playing at being cats

it is one of the best ways to learn about space, their bodies, social relationships and assessing risks and safety. Having a safe space to do it and an adult nearby will help.

### Activity

Think about how much time children are given in your setting to move about *freely* in the outdoor and indoor environment. If you work with babies, are they free to kick and wriggle on the floor on their backs and tummies, attentively watched over by staff? Is the environment set up to encourage toddlers to try out their newly developing gross motor skills? Can 2- to 5-year-olds get involved in vigorous physical activity? How are children with physical disabilities supported to join in? How do you encourage children who are reluctant to participate in this kind of activity?

## Fine motor skills

It takes quite a few months for a baby to develop accuracy in seeing something and being able to grasp it successfully. This is the beginning of hand–eye coordination. A few more months are needed before being able to move the object in exactly the way the baby intended. Large muscles develop ahead of fine motor skills and it all takes time. One skill builds on another and often the child will revert to using a former but more fully developed skill. It may take considerable time for a child to develop and always use the same effective grasp of a drawing implement or scissors. Chunky crayons, pens or pencils are easier for children at first. Most importantly, physical activity, preferably outside, where children can freely use their whole bodies for a wide range of movements, their arms as well as their legs, is essential in developing fine motor skills.

## Health and self-care

The second aspect of physical development highlighted in the EYFS is about keeping healthy, being aware of how to keep healthy and to care for oneself. The early learning goal associated with this aspect of learning shows high expectations of children's understanding: "Children know the importance for good health of physical exercise, and a healthy diet, and talk about ways to keep healthy and safe" (EYFS, 2012). This is an early learning goal for children to achieve by the end of the reception year, when most children are 5 years old. But it sounds a very tall order for young children, especially when there is so much concern that as a nation our diets are not very healthy and many of us do not exercise in anything like the amount we should.

So there is an urgent need for us to make sure that we are modelling how to keep healthy to the children, giving them plenty of opportunity for free physical play, fresh air and a healthy diet – and supporting parents to do this too. As we do so we need to be talking to the children about why physical activity, fresh air outdoors, a healthy diet and basic hygiene, such as cleaning teeth and washing hands, are important.

For babies and toddlers, health and self-care is about the way *we* look after *them*. The EYFS Statutory Framework places requirements on providers to ensure children's health needs are well catered for. For example,

"The provider must promote the good health of the children attending the setting."

"Where children are provided with meals, snacks and drinks, they must be healthy, balanced and nutritious."

"Fresh drinking water must be available and accessible at all times."

"Providers must provide access to an outdoor play area or, if that is not possible, must ensure that outdoor activities are planned and taken on a *daily* basis."

(EYFS Statutory Framework, 2012)

Promoting health for babies and young children means many conversations with parents about eating and care routines at home, so that there is continuity for babies and children between the setting and home.

## Looking at children:
## What do we see?

### Veronica, age 10 months

Veronica started in the nursery setting when she was 8 months old, two days per week. At 10 months she is competent at sitting up independently and can swivel herself round if something attracts her, such as a noise behind her. She stretches out for things that attract her attention and are just within reach. She is beginning to work out the position she needs to get herself into to crawl. In Figure 11.4a we can see her sitting, poised.

Veronica has noticed an object of interest (a board book) and is preparing to move to it.

She manages to get into the crawling position on hands and knees, by tipping forward and tucking one leg under her. She slowly makes her way to the book (see Figure 11.4b).

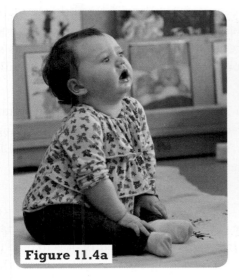

Figure 11.4a

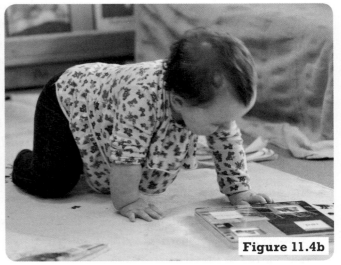

Figure 11.4b

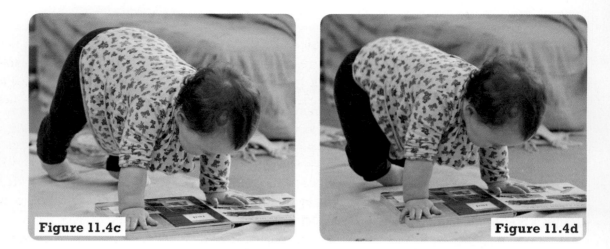

Figure 11.4c

Figure 11.4d

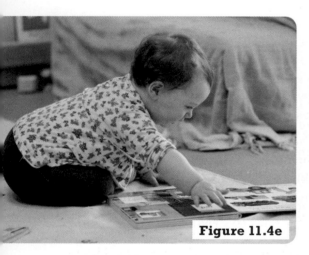

Figure 11.4e

The book is within reach. Now she wants to sit up again so she can free up her hands. She rises off her knees and balances on tiptoes and hands (see Figure 11.4c). One leg is curled forward under her (see Figure 11.4d). As she prepares to sit again in the new position, she frees up her hands to grasp the book – success!

## What have we found out?

Being able to move forward in this way is new to Veronica. It is an exciting development, allowing her to explore space and to move to objects that previously would have remained out of reach unless an adult or an older child had noticed what she wanted. To change from sitting immobile to crawling requires a great deal of thinking, working out how to move each part of the body, as well as using feet and fingers to grip and balance. As she coordinated her movements she independently achieved her goal – getting to the book and sitting back down in a new position to explore it with her hands.

We see Veronica developing her *physical skills*, both gross motor skills controlling her limbs, and small movements such as using her hands and feet, as well as fine motor skills – her finger control – to grasp the book. We also see *personal, social and emotional development* (PSED), developing confidence through successfully achieving her goal.

## Wilfred, age 3 years

Wilfred is beginning to use tools and decides to take part in a cutting activity. He picks up the scissors in both hands and begins to snip the paper. His key person shows him how to hold the scissors in one hand, where to put his thumb and fingers. He manages to control the scissors like this and continues to snip. "Look I did it," he says. Every now and then he reverts to using both hands to pull the scissors open, but goes back to trying it with one hand again when prompted. He concentrates hard on the activity of cutting.

## What have we found out?

Wilfred's growing hand–eye coordination and physical strength have helped him use a new tool: scissors. He knows how the tool works, but it is still easier for him at this early stage to hold the scissors in two hands to open and close. It may take a while for strength and technique to develop using just one hand. As we see in the observation, he returns to using two hands, which is still easier for him.

The adult-led activity is a very helpful one for learning to cut. The purpose of the activity is to use scissors. The children are not expected to cut anything out, but just to explore, play and practise. The paper was unwanted circulars, so that good quality paper was not wasted. In planning what next for Wilfred, his key person is very aware he needs more experience in learning how to use scissors, so more activities like this are needed. She decides that using scissors for other purposes, such as cutting dough or cutting ingredients in a cooking activity, will be helpful for him.

## What the experts say
### Importance of movement for healthy brain development

Sally Goddard Blythe is an expert in neurophysiological development and the author of several books for early years professionals and parents on child development, particularly physical development. Her books point out the importance of movement in supporting all learning, and the need for practitioners and parents to be aware of the impact on children's health and well-being when not enough opportunities to move freely are available. She promotes a whole body approach to learning, integrating the use of senses, thinking, movement, music and play. Music features strongly in her work. For example, much of her book, *The Genius of Natural Childhood* (Goddard Blythe, 2011), is devoted to rhymes, songs, action stories and games for babies to 5-year-olds, with clear instructions on the actions to use. It also provides a clear analysis of children's physical development and how to support it throughout the age range.

As a specialist she is well aware that some children need additional help in their physical development, and the importance of early diagnosis to ensure the right support is provided in a way that is fun and helps the children to learn.

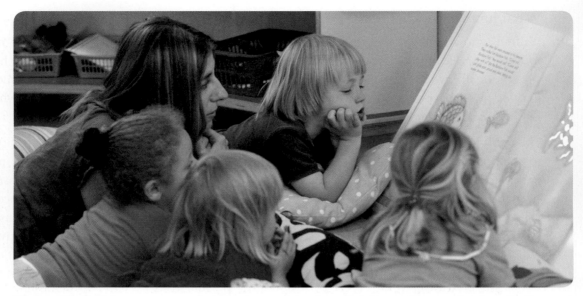

**Figure 11.5** Make sure you read stories in a variety of comfortable positions – a book on the floor while you and the children lie on your tummies is often the best way.

## JABADAO: Developmental Movement Play

In 2002, JABADAO, a charity set up in the mid 1980s to support the development of "a more wholehearted way of life", began a ten-year early years project – Developmental Movement Play. The project has involved groups of early years practitioners from a variety of settings to develop movement play. The project was set up because of the increasing awareness at JABADAO of the need to develop the understanding of early years practitioners about the importance of movement in children's learning and their confidence in supporting this. It began with training for the practitioners involved, who were then asked to develop an aspect of Developmental Movement Play in their setting.

The results have been very positive in increasing practitioner confidence and understanding: "movement is now seen as an underpinning for all development and learning, not just Physical Development" (JABADAO, 2009). The practitioners significantly increased the amount of movement play for the children in their settings, with more opportunities for spontaneous movement play, as well as better-run adult-led sessions. For example, most practitioners were able to develop a dedicated indoor space for movement play, as well as further developing their outdoor space. They increased the amount of floor space available and removed tables, so that children of all ages could spend more time working on the floor. Levels of well-being and involvement rose as a result.

The beneficial effects showed across all areas of learning and also resulted in a noticeable impact on children's levels of well-being and involvement. "Children learn just as well and sometimes better when adults control their (the children's) bodies less" (JABADAO, 2009). In addition, the increased understanding and confidence of the practitioners has meant that they were better at communicating the importance of movement in learning to parents too. You can find out more on the JABADAO website (www.jabadao.org).

# Effective practice:
## What do we need to do?

The EYFS 2012 has helped us to think again about how we support children's physical development and to make it a priority. As you think about effective practice, it is important to reflect on what you provide now and whether you are enabling all children to be physically active frequently enough to support their health and all other learning. It is not just theory or the EYFS that tells us being physically active and prioritising physical development is essential, but the children themselves indicate this to us all the time. In researching for my previous books I visited many schools and nursery settings. The practitioners and I talked to the children of 3, 4 and 5 years about their own learning. We asked them what was most important to them and what they wanted to learn next. Interestingly, the children's ideas of what was significant and what they wanted to learn next were most frequently physical skills (Hutchin, 2004, 2007).

Remember that things that do not cost money, or are very cheap, are often the best and the most interesting to the children. Providing for physical development often just means using the resources you have in new, creative and innovative ways. The list of child-initiated activities that help to develop both gross and fine motor skills, as well as balance, is almost endless!

## Moving and handling

- Provide the necessary support including accessibility for children and parents with physical disabilities so that they can participate fully in all that is provided.
- Have fun with the children. Joining in is important. You can encourage the less confident children to have a go and increase their enjoyment as you model being active to all the children.
- Give children time and space to try things out. It is all too easy to do things *for* the children! Without allowing children to become frustrated, help them by talking to them about what they are doing. Show interest and encouragement, sometimes suggesting trying another way, rather than doing it for them. This goes for all physical activities, whether it is about gross motor skills and movement or fine motor skills or self-care skills.
- Talk with parents about what you provide to support children's physical development and why. Talk with them about exercise and developing gross motor skills, for example the importance of developing their upper body and arm muscles, to support the development of fine motor skills.

### Freedom to play outside

- Wear the right clothing. Remember there is no such thing as bad weather, only bad clothing!
- Provide plenty of time for creative movement play outside. Ensure your environment is set up in a creative way that allows enough space for children to move freely and sometimes fast. A plank, tree trunk or wooden beam on the ground can encourage balancing. Is there a soft enough space (for example, a grassed area) where children can enjoy rough and tumble play without interrupting the play of others?

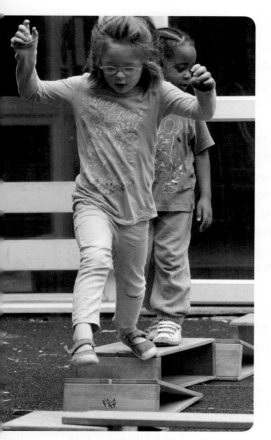

**Figure 11.6** Children can create their own obstacle courses

- Provide interesting opportunities for climbing and clambering. If you are in a setting that only has fixed climbing equipment, try to set up other opportunities for climbing and clambering, such as creating a changeable obstacle course. A table can make a tunnel, car tyres can become stepping stones. For babies, make sure there are different textured surfaces for crawling on – and of course, as for all children, that the area is hazard-free.
- Observe the children to make sure that your physical activities are challenging enough for them. Think of ways of extending their skills with the use of small equipment, such as balls to kick, throw or hit.

## Freedom to play indoors

- Plan for tummy time. Encourage babies and young children to spend time playing on their tummies. Some may need help to feel comfortable on their tummies – a rolled blanket to lie on may help, and for immobile babies, interesting, safe objects within reach.
- Think about your floor space. The JABADAO Developmental Movement Play project highlighted the need for a free movement space inside, as well as space and encouragement for movement outdoors. Think about how to free up some space for free movement and encourage children to use it for a range of movement on the floor, such as rolling, crawling, tilting, falling and jumping.

### Activity

#### Planning a space for movement and encouraging children to use it

Do you have too many tables and other furniture inside to allow room for a movement space? Find out more about why being able to move the body freely is so important to young children (see Further reading and references and Useful websites at the end of the chapter), and talk to your colleagues about how a space could be freed up in your setting and children encouraged to use it.

- Play games that encourage mobile toddlers and young children to move in creative ways, such as Follow my leader or Simon says. Provide the children with interesting movements they can try, perhaps with a theme such as gliding, slithering, tiny or giant movements, and then encourage the children to take turns at being the leader. Moving to a wide range of musical styles is important too, changing movements according to the rhythm.

### Fine motor skills

- Support the development of arm muscles, for example with bean bags to throw and shuttle cocks and lightweight balls to bat. Tying these to a tree branch or beam from the rain shelter (in a safe space, dedicated to this activity) will help children to develop their arm muscles. This in turn will help the development of fine motor skills. Use scarves and ribbons to twirl and dance with.

- Provide a range of opportunities to develop fine motor skills through child-initiated activities and planned activities. All the techniques used with malleable materials, such as clay or play dough, without tools will help develop fine motor skills – pinching, rolling, pulling, shaping and squashing.

- Help children learn how to hold tools. Using malleable materials with tools will help with children's ability to hold tools. Chubby crayons and pens will help children to develop strength to hold and manipulate them for mark-making. Tweezers for picking up small items help develop pincer grip, as will small pipettes with water, laces for threading beads and pegboards. A great activity seen in one setting was setting out a large tray of buttons, small stones and pretend gemstones, with a variety of real, small money purses with different closures. Another was the provision of a water tray with buttons and small stones with ladles and teaspoons. (See photos in Chapter 3.)

## Health and self-care

- Plan cooking activities with healthy recipes. Make sure that most of the cooking you do with children is around healthy foods and encourage them to taste and try. If they are not keen, sometimes seeing others try will encourage them. Where possible, plant vegetables in your outdoor area so that children can grow and harvest their own vegetables and fruit.

- Talk with children about their bodies and the changes that take place, for example, how they may sweat and feel hot when exercising, how they feel when they are hungry or thirsty, as well as about the kinds of foods that are healthy. Stories and books can be the basis for all sorts of interesting discussions on healthy living.

### Activity

#### Healthy eating

Make some simple recipe cards with the children, showing the healthy recipes you make together with them step by step. Illustrate each step with a photograph, so that the words match the picture. Making it into a small home-made book, putting each step on a separate page, will help children to understand the step-by-step approach as they turn the pages. Make similar illustrated recipe cards (perhaps the full recipe on one page) for parents too, so they can try it at home with their child – this could be a good fund-raiser! Make use of parents' own simple recipe ideas – and help to celebrate food from different cultures in the process.

## Case study: Woodlands Park: Growing healthy food in the garden

At Woodlands Park Nursery School and Children's Centre a few years, ago the parents using the Children's Centre wanted to learn how to garden with their children. The Centre helped by setting up a Gardening Club for parents and it is now run by one of the parents. A small group of children from the school also attend the Gardening Club every week. Then a new development was suggested for the nursery school children: why not have their own vegetable patch too, to look after themselves with the help and advice of the Gardening Club. Decisions had to be made about where it would be, how large and how to do it. It was agreed that raised beds would be best for the vegetables, and easiest for the children to be most involved. The job was done and the beds were ready for planting in March. They planted all sorts – potatoes, carrots, spinach, onions – and it all grew beautifully. By July the harvesting of juicy little carrots and green, green lettuce had begun. And the children had been involved all the way through – the vegetables were never short of water! Even though the juicy carrots were more popular, when we took these photographs most of the children were ready to at least try eating lettuce!

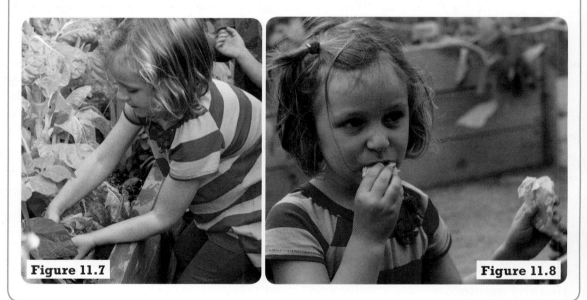

**Figure 11.7**  **Figure 11.8**

## Chapter summary

This chapter will have helped you:
➤ understand the importance of physical development to children's learning and general health and well-being
➤ find out what some experts have to say about physical development and how best to help children
➤ reflect on the practice in your own setting and how to improve your support for the children and the parents.

# Further reading and references

Bruce, T., Meggitt, C. and Grenier, J. (2010) *Childcare and Education*, Hodder Education, London (For more on the sequence of physical development and useful guidelines for practitioners see pp.130–5)

Evangelou, M., Sylva, K., Kyriacou, M., Wild, M. and Glenny, G. (2009) 'Early Years Learning and Development: Literature Review', DCSF Research Report RR176. Available to download from: www.education.gov.uk/publications/RSG/publicationDetail/Page1/DCSF-RR176

Goddard Blythe, S. (2005) *The Well Balanced Child: Movement and Early Learning*, Hawthorn Press, Stroud

Goddard Blythe, S. (2011) *The Genius of Natural Childhood: Secrets of Thriving Children*, Hawthorn Press, Stroud

Greenland, P. (2009) 'Physical Development' in *Early Childhood: A Guide for Students*, Bruce, T. (ed.), Sage Publications, London

Hutchin, V. (2004) *Observing and Assessing for the Foundation Stage Profile*, Hodder Education, London

Hutchin, V. (2007) *Supporting Every Child's Learning in the EYFS*, Hodder Education, London

Ouvry, M. (2003) Exercising Muscles and Minds, National Children's Bureau, London

School Food Trust (2012) 'Voluntary Food and Drink Guidelines for Early Years Settings in England – A Practical Guide'. Available to download from: www.schoolfoodtrust.org.uk/eatbetterstartbetter/practicalguide

Tickell, C. (2011) *The Early Years: Foundations for Life, Health and Learning*. An Independent Report on the Early Years Foundation Stage to Her Majesty's Government, Annex 9, p.92. Available to download from: www.education.gov.uk

White, J. (2007) *Playing and Learning Outdoors: Making Provision for High Quality Experiences in the Outdoor Environment*, The Nursery World/Routledge Essential Guides for Early Years Practitioners, Routledge, Abingdon

## Useful websites

JABADAO Developmental Movement Play: www.jabadao.org

Sally Goddard Blythe: www.sallygoddardblythe.co.uk

Interview with Sally Goddard Blythe: http://instantteleseminar.com/?eventid=21409257

School Food Trust: www.schoolfoodtrust.org.uk

# Section 4: Learning and Development Part 2: The specific areas of learning

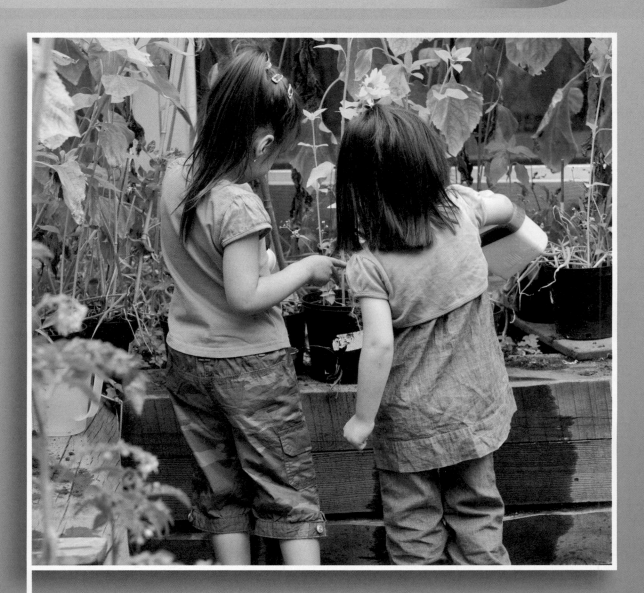

The revised EYFS has designated four areas of learning as specific:

Chapter 12: Literacy

Chapter 13: Mathematics

Chapter 14: Understanding the world

Chapter 15: Expressive arts and design.

# Chapter 12

# Literacy

## In this chapter we will be looking at:

➤ what this EYFS specific area of learning, Literacy, covers

➤ some observations of children developing interest and skills in reading and writing

➤ what an expert in early literacy has to say

➤ what we can do to ensure our practice is effective in supporting children's early literacy development.

## Introduction

All the settings featured in this book make books and stories a high priority. Children, from babies upwards, ask for books to be read to them all the time. A member of staff is always on hand to read a story or look through a book with a child, and often parents are available too. There are well used and inviting book areas displaying a range of books to cater for the children's tastes and interests. Baskets of story, information, poetry and rhyme books are kept in every area inside and in sheltered spots outside too. Story props and sacks are also available. Because the practitioners are so tuned in to the importance of reading, this has a real impact on children's all-round development, as well as their enthusiasm for talking about books, being read to and developing early literacy skills.

### The EYFS specific area of learning, Literacy, tells us:

"Literacy development involves encouraging children to link sounds and letters and to begin to read and write. Children must be given access to a wide range of reading materials – books, poems, and other written materials, to ignite their interest."

(EYFS Statutory Framework, 2012)

Literacy is a specific area of learning, covering the early skills, knowledge and understanding that children need as they progress towards mastering the complex skills of reading and writing. It is about how we "encourage" children and, as the Statutory Framework tells us, "ignite their interests" in learning to read and write. If we are enthusiastic and provide babies and children with opportunities to experience the wonderful world of books, stories, poems and rhymes by making it fun, children will be enthused too. They will *want* to pick up books to browse through and retell, and, so long as our enjoyment and enthusiasm continue, they will become avid readers in their later years, developing a lifelong love of books. We also want them to grow into adults who enjoy writing for pleasure, as well as using writing for functional purposes in their daily lives. By giving children plenty of opportunities to make marks in the earliest years, by appreciating their early attempts at writing and acting as scribes, writing down for them the messages they want us to write, we will help them to become competent, creative writers. Some children will need to learn alternative systems for reading and writing, such as Braille.

## What is this specific area of learning about?

Literacy is necessary to function successfully in the world. Being literate makes all the difference to children's "chances of social acceptability, worthwhile employment, extended educational opportunities and success" (Whitehead, 2009). To become literate children need to learn specific skills, knowledge and understanding. This learning is *dependent on* and *underpinned by* children's development in the prime areas of learning, particularly communication and language. In the Literacy area of learning, the EYFS 2012 highlights two aspects:

- **Reading**
- **Writing.**

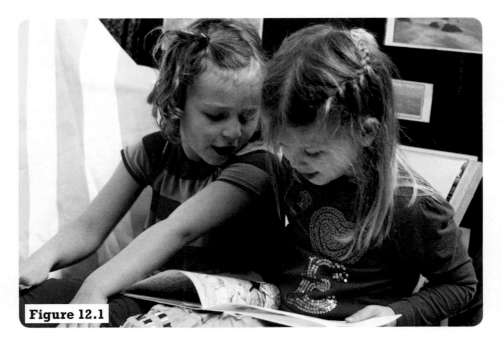

**Figure 12.1**

# Learning to read

## Reading for meaning

The process of reading involves:

- knowing that the marks on the page (the text) convey a message, wanting to know what that message is and understanding it – we often call this comprehension
- knowing how to de-code groups of symbols – this is often called word recognition and depends on the child's knowledge of phonics.

Phonics enables new readers to de-code written words by sounding out the spoken and written units within words. But reading is not just about de-coding the writing; it is about the meaning the writing conveys. Reading stories frequently to children, using books for information and talking about the signs around in the environment helps them to understand that the marks (writing) have a meaning. Children develop a deep interest in books and stories if they are read to frequently, given opportunities to look at books independently and become absorbed in retelling the stories to themselves. Gradually, as children seem to be ready for it, we need to draw their attention to the print.

Reading the pictures is an important part of learning to read, and in children's books, the pictures often tell the story as well as illustrate it. A good story leads children to want to know more and predict what might happen next – an important skill. Both of these processes are great ways to get the children to begin to take note of the print. As they talk about the pictures and make guesses about what might happen next, you can point to the words and say the initial letter sounds or, in texts where this works, you might leave a space so that they can guess the word that rhymes with the end of the previous sentence.

## Activity

Reflecting on your books:

1 Check through the books you have in your setting. Are they invitingly displayed and in good condition? Do they celebrate diversity? (See Activities in Chapter 1.)

2 Do you have a range of books to cater for all the children's interests? Check if you have the following:

- a wide range of different storybooks, from fun and scary tales (age-appropriate of course!) to warm and friendly ones
- poems and rhymes
- information books on topics likely to interest the children.

3 Are the books placed around your provision in different areas, inside and outside, to ignite children's interests?

4 How often do you change the books so that there is variety while ensuring that favourite books are always available?

### Talking about it

Making plenty of time to talk about the books, stories or the print in the environment around us is important. Talking about what they notice in the pictures helps children to focus on the detail – an important skill in learning to read. There is so much to talk about: the characters, the storyline, what happens next or what might have happened if ..., as well as the pictures.

### Rhythm and rhyme

The rhyme and rhythm in spoken language is also very important in learning to read, so frequently singing nursery rhymes and songs is essential. The rhythm helps children understand how speech is broken into words, and rhyme helps children to focus on the similar sound patterns in word endings.

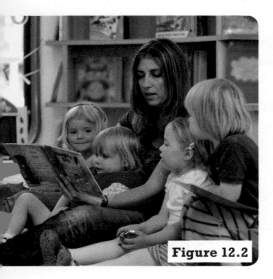

**Figure 12.2**

### Focus on the key words

When children are beginning to show interest in the print, the words that are stressed most are the first ones to show the children – such as the refrain or the word that is exaggerated. Children are always interested in reading and writing their own name. Usually the first letter of their name is the most significant to them at first, so a word beginning with the same letter is often a good place to start!

### Learning about letters and phonemes (phonics)

Providing alphabet friezes and books of all different kinds helps children get to know the letters of the alphabet. When they are showing interest in letters and the print around them they need to know the sounds the letters make – this is a very important part of learning to read. English does not have a simple pattern for letter–sound relationships: children need to know that some letters combine together to make a particular sound in a word and this is a very different sound from the sound the letter makes alone (for example, t with h makes a "th" sound.) Each sound is called a phoneme. There are 44 phonemes that we use in English.

As children learn to read, and once they are ready for it, usually in the reception class in school, they need to learn the phonemes. If you work with children who are 4 or 5 years old or more, it is important for you to know what the phonemes are and how to say them. When children are beginning to read for themselves, they need to blend the phonemes together to make words. English is a difficult language, because although there are many rules about how letters and phonemes fit together in words, the rules are often broken. Just think about the word "read" and how we say it differently depending on the tense. This makes us realise how complex it can be! Children also build up a memory of whole words, and this helps particularly with reading words that cannot be de-coded easily using phonics.

### Looking at a book together

Ask a child to look at a favourite storybook with you. Before you read the story, look through the book together. What does the child say? What seem to be the most important aspects to the child? Are they showing any interest in the print or pictures? If they are keen for you to get on with reading the story, read it to them and ask them afterwards about the parts they like best. If they are not interested at this time, choose another time and try again. Provide plenty of opportunities like this, however, for all the children.

## Writing

There are two skills children need as they learn to write:

1  deciding what to write (composition)
2  the physical act of writing it (transcription).

As handwriting is mostly about the physical skills children need to hold writing tools effectively, in the EYFS 2012 this is an aspect of physical development, fine motor skills.

### From making marks to writing

Children begin to make marks when they are babies – perhaps moving their hands or fingers backwards and forwards through spilled food or drink. Soon we begin to give them tools such as paintbrushes, pens and crayons to make marks, and later still they begin to tell us these marks have meanings – they become their creative representations. This is the beginning of representing things through drawing. As this development is taking place, children see adults writing and want to copy this idea. The first and most important thing they usually want to write is their own name. As they do this they bring the transcriptional and compositional aspects of writing together: they want to convey a message – their name – and attempt to make marks that look as close as they can make them to the letters of their name.

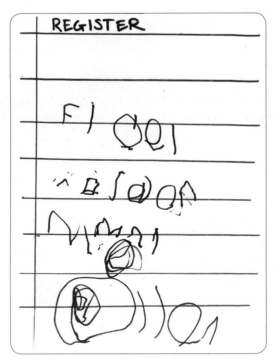

**Figure 12.3** Fidel, age 4 years 3 months, has written the names of some of the other children in his group, copied from their name cards

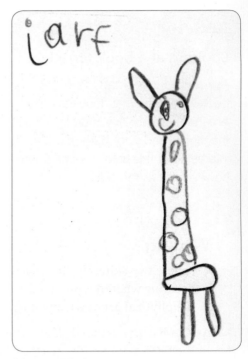

**Figure 12.4** Enya, aged just 5, has made a very plausible attempt at writing giraffe to label her drawing

## Composing what to write

We need to take care we do not concentrate on the transcriptional aspects of writing at the expense of the compositional. The most important aspect of writing is the message to be written – or composed – and this takes time to think up. We have to think about the topic and formulate the words in the right order before writing them down. Young children may be making writing-like marks for the pleasure of it and not have a message to write at first. One way to help children to understand that writing is all about having a message is writing down for them what they tell you about their drawings, paintings or models. Then, very soon, scribing what they dictate to us in other situations comes very naturally.

## Case study: Molly's dragon story

The physical aspect of writing is difficult for young children. Molly is one of the youngest children in the reception class. The teacher asked the children to draw their stories about dragons and to dictate the words to a member of staff. Children were able to concentrate on their creative writing and, as a result, every story in the class was exciting and different.

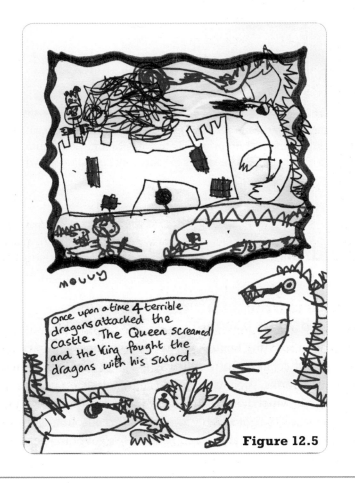

MOLLY

Once upon a time 4 terrible dragons attacked the Castle. The Queen screamed and the King fought the dragons with his sword.

**Figure 12.5**

## Making the link between letters and sounds when writing

We call the way we write a phoneme a grapheme. When children are ready, usually, but not always, around the age of 5 years, they need support to learn about how to break words up (segment) into their component parts (phonemes) to write them (graphemes). If you see children's emergent writing when they are beginning to grasp the correspondence between phonemes and graphemes, you will notice that they are making phonetically plausible attempts at writing words. They will also be beginning to write some simple, frequently used words from memory.

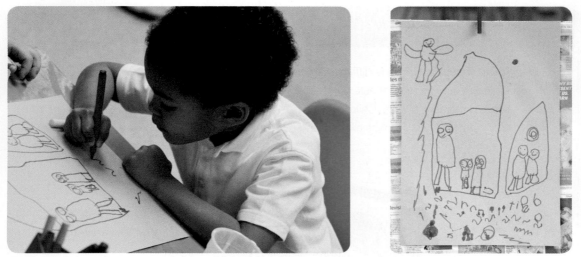

**Figure 12.6** This child came into the nursery this morning and immediately sat down to draw his story. Once he had completed his drawing he began to write about it. No one asked him to do this; he had his own ideas, was willing to have a go, using what he knows to represent his ideas. His writing says: 'All the monsters live in the cave'.

## Looking at children:
## What do we see?

### Zeinaddine, age 3 years 6 months

Zeinaddine was new to learning English when he started in the nursery school six months ago. His understanding and speaking of English is growing rapidly. He has become increasingly interested in favourite books, such as *The Gruffalo* by Julia Donaldson. On this occasion, as he looks through the book, which has been read to him on many previous occasions, he says: "It's a Gruffalo. He's a monster. He's got wobbly knees and turned-out toes and a mouse. The Gruffalo licked the mouse. He picked his tail up and licked. He's got orange eyes and a black tongue."

### What have we found out?

At 3 years 6 months Zeinaddine is able to narrate parts of the story through reading the pictures and remembering some of the repeated refrains. It is possible that, reading the pictures, the snake slithering away is the tail he is referring to, and he associates the Gruffalo's tongue pictured on the page before as licking the tail. Other observations of Zeinaddine at this time show his interest in other aspects of early literacy: he loves to sing songs, enjoys mark-making and is beginning to want to write his name.

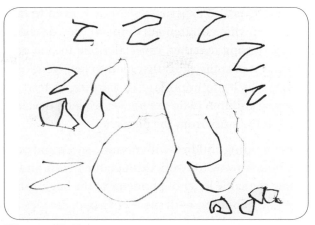

**Figure 12.7** Zeinaddine's name writing

### Annie, 3 years 7 months

Annie joins her key person at the writing table, takes a chunky felt-tip and begins to make marks on the small whiteboard in front of her. Her key person is involved with other children, but when she turns to Annie she sees she has written "Anni" and attempted to make an "e". She says: "Wow Annie, what have you written?"

Annie: "My mummy showed me how to do my name," and she pointed to the letters saying "A-n-n".

Her key person offered to show her how to do an "e".

Annie: "I don't want you to help me!"

After this she writes the letter A shape all around the edge of the paper but without the horizontal line across the middle. "These are As," she says.

Key person: "Where are the lines to cross them?"

Annie: "I do it after."

Then she went back to put the lines across most of the As.

### What did we find out?

Annie has chosen to write her name and to practise writing the initial letter; nobody has asked her to do this. Her mother has helped her by showing her how to make the letter shapes. She also knows the names of the letters in her name and she is pleased about her new skill. On seeing this Learning Story with photographs of Annie writing, her mother was thrilled: "I am amazed she has started to write her name. It's fabulous."

## What the experts say
### Helping children to become literate

Marian Whitehead's work on language and literacy is well known through her many books and articles. In her work she describes the processes children need to develop and gives practical advice on the sorts of activities and experiences children need to become literate. Her writing is full of useful examples of what children are doing as they develop literacy skills. She writes about the importance of reading together, especially one to one or in small groups. She also writes about the importance of some skills that tend to get overlooked, such as when children are memorising the text, which are important to learning to read (Whitehead, 2009). Other important skills that young children (who are not yet readers) develop must not be overlooked, such as being able to retell the story from the pictures.

She believes too that surrounding children with rhymes, songs and poems will help them to gain important knowledge about how words work through the rhyme and rhythm in the language, as well as alliteration (using the same letter or phoneme at the beginning of the word). She stresses the importance of providing children with plenty of opportunities and encouragement to talk about books and the print they see around them that they may show interest in.

## Effective practice:
## What do we need to do?

### Reading
- Have lots of conversations with children – the size of children's vocabulary has an impact on their ability to read in later years. The only way of extending vocabulary in the early years is through talk.
- Sing rhymes and songs daily with babies, toddlers and young children. Make sure you sing the words clearly so children know what they are.
- Read plenty of storybooks, poems and rhymes and information books to babies and children.

### Activity

#### Reading for pleasure
How often are books shared with children one to one or in a very small group in your setting? Over the course of two days (ideally not two consecutive days), keep a tally of how often you and other staff read books to groups of up to four or five children during the session. Make a note of which children get this quality literacy time and which children do not. Are some children missing out? How can you encourage children who may be missing out? Is it about finding the right time of day for them, or perhaps your books do not cater for their interests?

- Have a group of favourite books and stories to read and reread frequently and use them as the basis for planned activities – acting out the story, retelling it in a new way, making displays about it, helping children to make their own versions of the book.
- Make time to talk about the book when reading one to one or in a very small group. Focus on what interests the children and sometimes point out features of the print, particularly words that have a particular importance to the story.

- Make sure children know what the words on your displays say. Draw children's attention to the print around them.
- Play listening games to support children's developing listening skills. This will help them tune their ears to the sounds within words that are needed for reading and writing.
- Ensure all children can be involved in the full range of literacy experiences with the support and additional aids they may need, including signing and learning to read Braille, as appropriate.

## Writing

Many of the points for effective practice in reading also help to develop writing skills.
- Model writing for a purpose to the children, by writing your own lists, notes, notices and messages in front of them. Tell them what you are writing as you do it.

For children over 2 years:
- Provide plenty of opportunities and reasons to make meaningful marks, for example, shopping lists, registers, messages and appointments in role play.
- Encourage children to make marks by showing interest in the marks they make, listening carefully to them when they tell you about their marks.
- Make name cards for the children that they can take with them to different areas of the setting to use to help them write their names.
- Make books with the children, for example about the children themselves, about outings and children's favourite play scenarios.
- Make notices with the children, for example notices for parents or reminders to children to put the tops on the pens and to hang up their coats.

### Activity

### Writing for a purpose

There are lots of reasons to write messages with the children. Find a reason for making a book with the children – it could be based around a play theme, such as firefighters, superhero favourites, scary monsters or a favourite teddy. It could be about an outing they have been on. Illustrations may be photographs or the children's own drawings, but explain to the children that the book will need some writing too. Ask them what you should write and encourage children to do their own mark-making and writing too.

- Have equipment for writing everywhere – various sizes of clipboards, chalkboards, notepads, office areas and keyboards.
- Encourage children to tell you their stories and act as a scribe for them. See the Case study of Molly's dragon story on page 177.

## Case study: St Anne's Nursery School and Children's Centre: The Bilingual Book Club

At this nursery school and Children's Centre in London, all children are invited to take a book home every day. They can enjoy their favourite books at home with their families and change the book for another one as often as they like. Parents and practitioners work together to encourage children's enthusiasm for books and reading and it works really well.

At the school usually around 50 per cent of the children are learning English as an additional language, with between 15 and 20 different home languages. To cater for this the school created a Bilingual Book Club, which includes bilingual books in every language of the school's population. Every week the parents of the children learning English as an additional language bring their children to choose a book in their first language to borrow. The impact has been immense, with highly positive feedback from parents. One parent commented that as a result of the book club, the whole family is now learning to read in their first language, which they speak but had never learned to read.

For all the children in the school there are bilingual story sessions too, where a parent who speaks a language other than English is invited to read to a group of children. As all children are invited to attend; they are given the experience of hearing a language other than English.

## Chapter summary

This chapter will have helped you:
➤ understand more about how children learn to read and write
➤ reflect on what you can do to support them in the early stages of learning to read and write.

## Further reading and references

Donaldson, J. (1999) *The Gruffalo*, Macmillan Children's Books, London

Whitehead, M.R. (2009) *Supporting Language and Literacy Development in the Early Years* (2nd edn), Open University Press/McGraw-Hill, London

Whitehead, M.R. (2010) *Language and Literacy in the Early Years, 0–7*, Sage Publications, London

# Chapter 13

# Mathematics

## In this chapter we will be looking at:

➤ what this EYFS specific area of learning, Mathematics, covers

➤ some observations of children developing mathematical skills and understanding

➤ what some experts in children's early mathematical development have to say

➤ what we can do to ensure our practice is effective in supporting young children's mathematical development.

## Introduction

Emma is now just 2 years old. She loves saying numbers as she walks up the stairs. She can say numbers to 19 in Spanish, her first language and in English to 10 – the language she uses at her nursery. Everyone can tell she really enjoys doing it. She loves counting other things too – anything that is countable. She gets much of the number sequence right usually and will carry on saying numbers if someone starts this in the middle. If you say "seven" she will add "eight, nine, ten". Her counting is not always accurate – she may skip a number name or count the same stair or object twice – but it is a fun game and a great achievement, and she can switch from one language to the other as she does so! If you ask her how old she is she proudly tells you – in Spanish or in English – that she is 2 years old.

## The EYFS specific area of learning, Mathematics, tells us:

"Mathematics involves providing children with opportunities to develop and improve their skills in counting, using and understanding numbers, calculating simple addition and subtraction problems; and to describe shapes, spaces, and measures."

(EYFS Statutory Framework, 2012)

Over the last few years early years policy in England has renamed the area of learning now called Mathematics twice. For many years it was called Mathematical development, and then in the 2008 EYFS it became Problem solving, Reasoning and Numeracy (PSRN). In 2012 it changed to the name used for the curriculum area for older children: Mathematics. Much of the content has remained the same as before. However, calculating, which was previously a separate aspect, is now incorporated into numbers.

As a specific area of learning, mathematics is dependent on and underpinned by the prime areas of learning. Children's earliest encounters with mathematics are social ones – such as one for you, one for me. These encounters involve the child's physical development as she/he explores shape, space and measure, and sometimes number too, and all mathematics involves communicating ideas.

## What is this specific area of learning about?

The two aspects of Mathematics that are highlighted in the EYFS 2012 are:
- **numbers**
- **shape, space and measures.**

Mathematics in the EYFS is not just about being able to count accurately, know the names and properties of shapes or how things can be measured, although these are important concepts. It is about young children being interested in the mathematical aspects of the world around them and in solving simple, practical mathematical problems and developing a day-to-day mathematical vocabulary of number, shape, position, size and weight, for example. This is exciting learning, which starts very young. Well before Emma was 2 years, she was developing a great deal of mathematical awareness about her surroundings and using it in her everyday life.

One of the key messages from recent research on mathematics in the early years is that "beginning formal instruction at an early age does not improve subsequent mathematical achievement" (Evangelou *et al.*, 2009). This means a focus on the first-hand, practical, everyday experiences, and a problem-solving approach is essential.

### Mathematical language

A key element of mathematics is the mathematical language used in number and shape, space and measures, as well as problem solving. We use mathematical vocabulary all the time, but are often not aware of it. Children pick up this mathematical vocabulary in the normal course of day-to-day talk. If we only use words such as big and little, rather than long/short, wide/narrow, heavy/light, then children will only learn big and little, so we do need to be accurate in the terminology we use.

### Numbers

#### Recognising quantity and number

Research shows that babies as young as 5 months old are able to recognise how many without counting and can recognise the difference between sets of one, two or three objects. As soon as they can talk, words such as more are used frequently in all sorts of ways, such as in fun and games with others and with objects.

## Knowing number names

If number words are used and encouraged in the home or setting, for example through singing rhymes and songs and games, children will pick up this knowledge quickly. They may not be said in order at first or used for counting, but young children, like Emma, love to say numbers. Children of 3 and 4 years often love to talk about numbers, especially the number that is the personally significant one. When you are counting "1, 2, 3, 4" to a child, you will often hear them say: "I'm 4!" They also love big numbers, such as hundreds and millions.

## Counting

Counting means one-to-one correspondence between the spoken numeral and the object to be counted, even if the object cannot be seen. Learning one-to-one correspondence (to say one number for each object in order) takes time to establish in young children, and they need to start with small numbers, real objects and real purposes for counting. Board games appropriate to the ages of the children can provide opportunities to introduce counting as well as being great fun.

## Representing numbers

Children develop their own ways of representing numbers if they are encouraged to do so. This is an important part of developing understanding about number and should be encouraged in play, by providing drawing and writing materials for many play purposes – such as in role play, or playing games or turn taking with the wheel toys.

## Recognising written numerals

The first written numeral most children will recognise is their personal number – their age – particularly from 3 or 4 years onwards. Gradually, if numerals are readily available to touch, hold, play with and see, children will become familiar with them; but to understand what these symbols are means seeing them used in everyday situations, not being given lessons or worksheets.

## Using numbers to calculate

Number rhymes and songs help children to take away and add – in fact, in most of our number songs the numbers are taken away, helping children to learn about one less. There are many games that can help children learn to add one more. Helping children find their own number problems for real purposes, such as sharing things out between their key group or a group of friends, is important in making it relevant to them.

### Activity

During a half-day session at your setting, listen to how many times in the course of children's play and other self-chosen activities (for example, role play, sand and water, and physical play inside and outside) you hear children talk about numbers, quantities, size or shape. What sort of vocabulary are the children using? Are you aware of how often you use mathematical vocabulary too? If there is little mathematical language from the children, make sure you incorporate more into your conversations with them.

## Shape, space and measures

Young babies start to develop awareness of shape, space and pattern very early, as they begin to explore the world visually at first, and then with their hands, mouths and feet. A wide variety of real objects to explore, such as in a treasure basket or in heuristic play, gives them rich provision in which to experience three-dimensional shapes and all their properties, such as weight, length, whether something has corners, is spherical or cylindrical. As they explore, children become fascinated by piling up bricks and knocking them down, hiding objects inside or under other objects. They are exploring mathematical concepts of position, size, shape and space.

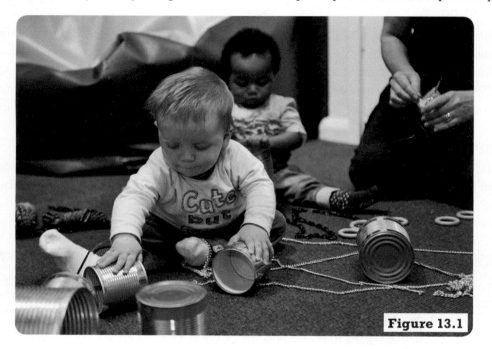

Figure 13.1

### Activity

As you watch a baby exploring objects in a treasure basket or a toddler engaged in heuristic play (see Chapter 8), work out how many different types of mathematical concepts are being explored – for example quantity, number, size or shape, or space. If you work with older children, watch some children playing with sand or water instead.

As children play we need to talk to them about what they are doing, and in the course of the conversations, introduce the relevant mathematical vocabulary, referring, for example, to the name of the shape they are exploring. This does not mean asking them closed questions, such as what shape it is or how many, but introducing the correct terms in the course of your own informal interactions.

Outdoor play on climbing equipment, with wheel toys or simply exploring the environment provides a wealth of opportunities to talk about shape, position and all kinds of measurement, such as speed, length, height and weight. Block play provides a wonderful opportunity for children to explore shape, space and measures. Pattern is a very important aspect of shape, space and measures. There is a wealth of opportunities to point out pattern to children as you work with them – in their creations as well as in clothing and in the environment around them, including paving, brickwork in walls and buildings, the sunlight through the trees or stones and leaves.

## Activity

Look at your outdoor area and think about how many opportunities there are for mathematical experiences and thinking. Is there provision for learning about numbers, counting, shape, space and measures? Are there opportunities for children to make mathematical marks, for example developing awareness of shape and space through chalking on the ground or painting with water? Check if there are enough opportunities to play games that provide purposes for mathematical mark-making, such as scoring in skittles or throwing balls into buckets.

# Looking at children:
## What do we see?

### Veronika, age 3 years 10 months

Hollow blocks are designed so that there a three different lengths: a quarter length, half and full length. Veronika was in the block area, fitting the hollow blocks together flat on the floor, so that no spaces were left. "I am making a stage," she said. When all the blocks were used up she found that she had a small gap in the middle, the size of the smallest block. "Where's the small one? There's usually a small one!"

As it could not be found, her key person helped her reorder some of them, but this made a gap at the edge. Looking at the gap, Veronika said: "There could be some steps here." She rushed off the find some foam blocks and placed them where the block was missing, testing them out to check they would work.

"Welcome to the Pantomime of Jingle Jangle! If you are going to see the show you will need a ticket!" She found a sheaf of tickets and gave them to her key person: "These are for sharing." She fetched some chairs, moving other obstacles out of the way to place them near the stage.

### What have we found out?

When Veronika's key person analysed this observation she realised how much learning was going on in this completely self-initiated play activity, especially the richness of the mathematical learning about shape, space and measure. Veronika is building on her knowledge about *shape and space* as she finds a problem to solve: how to fill a gap in her pattern. She shows awareness of the shapes and sizes of the blocks and uses the vocabulary of size too ("the small one"). She knows exactly what is missing and realises she can fill the gap adequately with another resource of similar dimensions (this requires *measurement*). All this is taking place in a self-initiated activity, with Veronika highly motivated to fulfil her aim – make a stage for the show.

### Fidel, age 5 years

Fidel is at the water tray, which has been set up with small ladles, spoons, little metal pans and buttons. He is with two boys, ladling up the buttons and pouring them into a saucepan, and he appears to be delighted by what he is doing.

Speaking to the younger boy opposite him, Fidel says: "Look I got a tiny baby one. Now I got three. This is like soup, it's like soup! …" [referring to ladle].

They continue counting as they scoop up the buttons. Other boy: "I've got nine … I've got nine again!" Fidel: "No, you haven't, you've got three! What have you caught? I've got three!"

### What have we found out?

This activity has been set up for children to explore the resources in ways of their own choosing. The interesting provision has drawn the children to play here. It is not specifically set up as a counting activity. Fidel chose to focus on number. He shows that he knows three just by looking. He is well aware of the difference between nine and three. As he was expressing his understanding of number, he was also fully absorbed in this playful self-chosen activity, bringing in his imaginative thinking ("it's like soup").

## What the experts say
### Encouraging young children's mathematical mark-making

Elizabeth Carruthers and Maulfry Worthington have researched young children's mathematical mark-making (which they call mathematical graphics) for many years and written extensively about it. They show us how children use their "graphical marks, symbols and representations" to explore and communicate their mathematical thinking. Their book, *Understanding Children's Mathematical Graphics: Beginnings in Play* (Carruthers and Worthington, 2011) includes a chapter on the deliberate scribbles of babies and the beginnings of graphical representations of toddlers and 2-year-olds. All their books are full of carefully analysed examples of children's mathematical graphics.

Mathematical graphics is not about how children write down or record their mathematics or sums once they have worked them out – the kind of recording usually expected in primary or secondary school with older children, but how young children *use* mark-making (graphics) to develop their thinking. Carruthers and Worthington note that whereas we often look for emergent writing in children's drawings and graphical representations, we tend to overlook their "mathematical graphics". They believe we need to take children's *informal* representations of mathematical thinking more seriously. They emphasise the importance of the:

*"environment, the sensitive interactions with children through co-constructing learning and scaffolding and the understanding that mathematics does not take place only in set adult-directed times but is threaded throughout the day within a culture of mathematical enquiry"*

(Carruthers and Worthington, 2011)

# Effective practice:
## What do we need to do?

When considering effective practice in mathematics in the early years, the first thing we need to do is look at ourselves: if you ask adults about how confident they are in mathematics, many will say it is not something they feel confident in or will even say they cannot do it! Yet young children are fascinated by patterns they see, excited by numbers and use their budding mathematics easily in their play – we need to notice it and celebrate it. There is potential for mathematical thinking in so many of the explorations, activities and investigations children get involved in every day. "Children can learn mathematics through play provided there is deliberate, thoughtful planning for and from children's interests, with long uninterrupted periods for them to play" (Carruthers and Worthington, 2011).

- Support parents by running practical workshops on mathematics in the early years. The case study at the end of this chapter is a good example of this.

- Make sure your environment, inside and outside, provides rich and interesting opportunities to develop all aspects of children's mathematical thinking. Look carefully at your resources: do they enable children to see the mathematical potential?

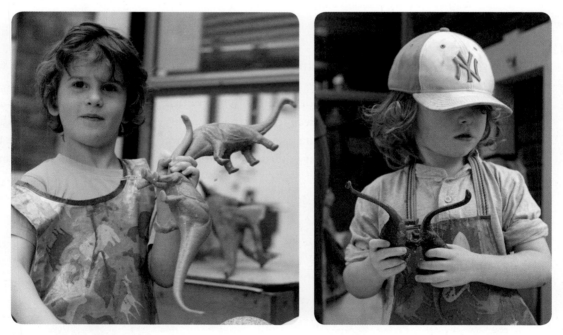

**Figure 13.2** These boys were playing together and the play depended on finding matching pairs of dinosaurs. Thinking about mathematical potential in resources is important.

- Remember that research shows that young children's mathematics learning is not about formal adult-led activities, but interacting with children informally, using the opportunities that arise in their play. These can be followed up in other ways, such as through conversation, playing games and providing some adult-led activities that tap into children's interests and are flexible enough to accommodate children's existing knowledge, skills and understanding.

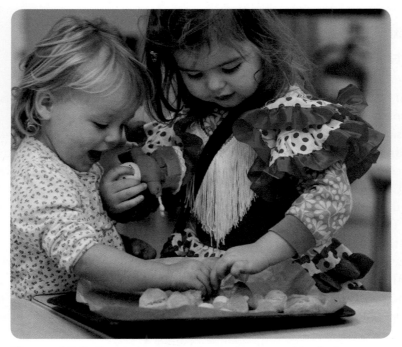

**Figure 13.3** Cooking can provide good opportunities for language and skills in mathematics

- Take a problem-solving approach, setting up investigations that you know the children will be interested in, using opportunities that arise to ask open-ended questions to spark off children's mathematical thinking. For example, when cutting up the fruit for a snack, ask the children involved: "How many pieces of banana do we need today?" Then some children can ask the others who wants banana and record the answers in their own ways. Use the appropriate mathematical language as you cut the fruit together – half, quarter, and so on.

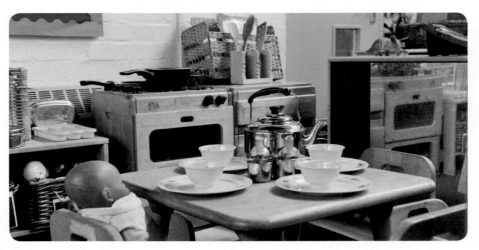

**Figure 13.4** Make sure the resources in the home corner match in number (four chairs, four cups, four plates, and so on)

- Encourage children to set their own problems. Model this by taking a problem-solving approach when problems arise, asking them to help you.
- Encourage children's mathematical graphics by providing a variety of tools, for example, have clipboards in every area, chalks to use on the ground, and an easel with large paper for scoring in games such as skittles.
- Make your own mathematical games, trails and tracks. Board games can very easily be made with children, based on their play themes, using dice or spinners and a piece of card for a board. On a larger scale, a giant-sized game can be chalked onto the hard surface, making stepping stones or running to a space with a particular number or pattern on it.
- Make use of tidy-up time to develop mathematical awareness. Store resources so children can see the mathematical potential as they tidy up, and make tidying up into a fun, challenging mathematical experience.

## Number

- Sing plenty of number songs and rhymes. Act them out with the children as characters and also use props (such as five frogs or ducks), so children can see the number. This will help children with English as an additional language to understand too.
- Use books and stories. Making up your own number stories where a character (teddy/doll) gets the counting wrong can be great fun, as the children correct the mistakes the character makes. Many stories have an element of mathematical thinking in them – often about number.
- Help children with counting by pointing to each item, saying the number as you do so (for example "1, 2, 3, 4, 5"). When you have come to the end of the items being counted, make a circular movement with your finger ("That's five altogether"). This helps young children pick up the difference between counting in order and the final number in the group.
- Play board games with children that are appropriate to their level of understanding. Even taking turns in these games is a mathematical concept in itself, counting and sharing out the pieces needed to play the game. Board games are often about number, but also incorporate other aspects of mathematics, such as pattern, shape, size.

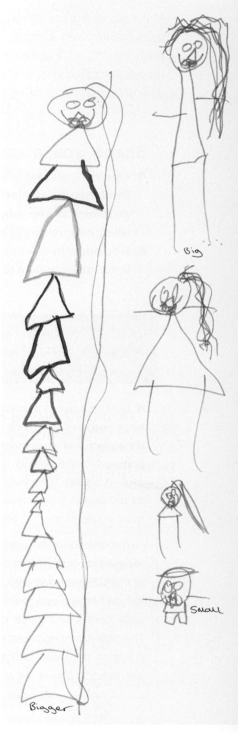

**Figure 13.5** Malak's drawing was her way of describing size differences (Hutchin, 2004)

## Shape, space and measures

■ Observe children involved in block and construction play. Then, when appropriate, get involved too, as a play partner. As you do so, introduce mathematical language, raise children's awareness of the properties of the shapes and encourage the children to take a problem-solving approach, by asking open-ended questions: "I wonder what would happen if …"

■ Find opportunities to measure things in real situations, for example needing a new rug in the book area, or when moving furniture around.

## Case study: St Anne's Nursery School and Children's Centre: Mathematics workshops for parents

At St Anne's Nursery School and Children's Centre the staff run a workshop for parents on mathematics every year, as part of their Family Learning Programme. The aim of the workshop is to develop parents' confidence and knowledge about mathematics and children's mathematical development, and it is very popular with the parents. There are two sessions: the first session is for the parents alone, while in the second session the parents and their children come together. In the first session there is plenty of time for discussion, for example about how children learn numeracy and the difference between knowing the number names and actually counting.

Two members of the staff team run the sessions, providing a wide variety of games and hands-on experiences that are used with the children in the school. Parents are encouraged to have a go at all of them. Explanation cards show parents what the children will be learning. There are also games that the staff have made, building on children's interests – for example, using cars or trains, skittles using water bottles, and songs, rhymes and stories. The emphasis is on games and activities that are no cost. The parents are encouraged to ask questions, with plenty of time for discussion about how to build on children's particular interests at home. In the second session the children join their parents, doing the activities and playing the games together.

## Chapter summary

This chapter will have helped you:
➤ understand more about how children learn about number and shape, space and measures
➤ reflect on what you can do to support children's learning in mathematics through the provision you make and how you respond to the children.

## Further reading and references

Carruthers, E. and Worthington, M. (2008) *Children's Mathematics: Making Marks, Making Meaning* (2nd edn.), Sage Publications, London

Carruthers, E. and Worthington, M. (2011) *Understanding Children's Mathematical Graphics: Beginnings in Play*, Open University Press/McGraw-Hill, London

Evangelou, M., Sylva, K., Kyriacou, M., Wild, M. and Glenny, G. (2009) 'Early Years Learning and Development: Literature Review', DCSF Research Report RR176. Available to download from: www.education.gov.uk/publications/RSG/publicationDetail/Page1/DCSF-RR176

Skinner, C. (2005) *Maths Outdoors*, BEAM Education, Cheltenham

Stevens, J. (2008) *Maths in Stories*, BEAM Education, Cheltenham

### Useful websites

Family Learning: www.familylearning.org.uk

# Chapter 14

# Understanding the world

## In this chapter we will be looking at:

➤ what this EYFS specific area of learning, Understanding the world, covers

➤ some observations of children developing their thinking and knowledge about the world around them

➤ how the Forest School approach is helping children's learning about the natural world

➤ some examples of what you can do to ensure your practice is effective in this area of learning.

## Introduction

A practitioner has placed a large map of the world on a table. A display is being created for the children, to help them understand about places in the world and how their small community links with other places. Some parents are gathered around with their children and with photographs of family members. There is an exciting buzz around the table. This has been going on at the beginning of the morning every day this week, involving different parents and their children, and will continue until every child's family is included.

There is also a photograph of every child, taken in the nursery. The parents are writing labels about who is in the photograph (grandmother, grandfather, uncle or aunt) and the country or town they live in. Emily's mother has a photograph of her grandmother and grandfather in Leeds and her other grandmother in Essex; Ryan's grandmother lives in London and his grandfather lives in St Lucia; Amir's aunt and uncle live in Pakistan, and his grandparents live in London. The parents point out to their children the places on the map where family members live.

When it goes on the wall the photographs will be placed around the map, with string linking the photographs to the places where they live and captions written under the photographs. The photographs of the children will be displayed too. The aim is to make sure everyone – children, their parents and visitors – get a sense of the setting's own community, helping the children's understanding of their world. It will go alongside the welcome poster that says "welcome" in all the different languages of the local community.

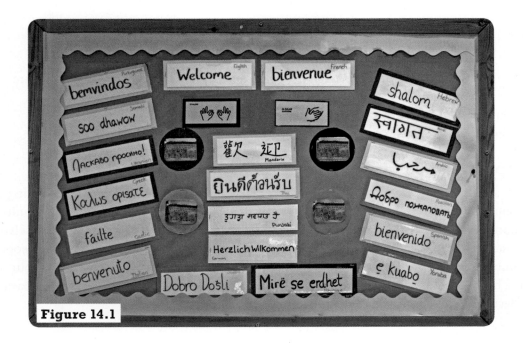

**Figure 14.1**

## The EYFS specific area of learning, Understanding the world, tells us:

"Understanding the world involves guiding children to make sense of their physical world and their community through opportunities to explore, observe and find out about people, places, technology and the environment."

(EYFS Statutory Framework, 2012)

This area of learning was previously called Knowledge and understanding of the world, and included wide-ranging aspects of learning and development. In the 2012 EYFS it was simplified to cover three main aspects of learning. It links closely with *how* children learn, finding things out by exploring and thinking critically (see Section 2, The characteristics of effective learning). Like the other specific areas of learning, Understanding the world is dependent on the prime areas of learning, in particular:

- making relationships (personal, social and emotional development)
- children's physical interactions with their surroundings, using their growing physical skills (physical development)
- interacting with others (communication and language).

It is also closely related to the other specific areas of learning, as children express their ideas and develop their thinking.

The three aspects of Understanding the world that are highlighted in the EYFS 2012 are:
- **People and communities**
- **The world**
- **Technology.**

## People and communities

The activity involving a map and photographs of relatives described at the beginning of the chapter helps children to develop a sense of themselves as part of a wider community – an important aspect of this area of learning. People and communities also relates closely to the principle and theme of EYFS discussed in Chapter 1. Children's learning about people and communities depends not only on relationships at home, but the *inclusive ethos* in your setting and how the similarities and differences between people are celebrated. Have a look back at the Effective practice section and Activity 2 in Chapter 1.

### Children's diverse experiences

Children's knowledge about people and communities begins at home within the family. They each come to early years settings with very different experiences of people outside their immediate family. For some, visits to the homes of other family members and friends are frequent. Here they will see various expectations and habits, cooking and food, which are different from those they see at home. These experiences broaden their personal views of the world. For other children, who may be far away from extended family and have few friends in the immediate neighbourhood, such experiences may be quite limited. Close relationships and regular communication with parents will help practitioners to build on children's individual experiences.

### Expanding children's awareness

Books and stories, particularly those where the setting of the story and the characters may be culturally different from the experiences of the children, will be very valuable in expanding children's knowledge and understanding. Songs and rhymes from other cultures and celebrating festivals will also help. Outings in the local community, such as shopping to buy ingredients for cooking or a visit to the local fire station, religious building or clinic, will help to expand the child's knowledge and awareness. Providing suitable resources from a range of cultures for the home corner, for example, will also expand children's awareness. Planned activities, such as cooking recipes from a range of cultures, are useful too – even more so if parents can be involved.

With support, children develop their awareness, understanding and acceptance of others. As their communication and language skills develop, and so long as practitioners and parents encourage them, they will be keen to share their own experiences, listen to others and discuss what they are finding out. This will help build a sense of identity, personal history and community.

Children's awareness and personal understanding of inclusion will be further developed by using signing, reading stories in children's first languages, putting signs up in Braille, for example.

## The world

What does this mean for babies and young children? Young children's curiosity and first-hand explorations help them find out about the natural world of mini beasts, animals and plants; the properties of materials such as water and sand; the changes that take place as ingredients are mixed together in cooking; the places and spaces around them and further afield; and how things work. Providing maps and activities, such as the one described at the beginning of the chapter, will help develop children's awareness of places in the world, and even if families do not come from far afield, they can locate places where relations live or where they go on holiday.

Supporting children to explore the world is a core aspect of the practitioner's role in an early years setting. The opportunities to provide a wide range of appropriate activities and learning experiences that will enthuse and motivate the children and babies to want to find out for themselves are endless. Planning safe and interesting possibilities to provide for the children is exciting as we nurture their curiosity and encourage them to question and enquire.

The "importance of inquiry-based approaches" in supporting the development of children's scientific thinking was wholeheartedly endorsed by the review of the research prepared for the revised EYFS 2012. The review goes further than taking an investigative approach: practitioners need to "convey to children the importance of not just 'what happens' or 'how it happens' but 'why it happens'" (Evangelou *et al.*, 2009). We need to be encouraging children to ask us "why" questions. Interestingly, research shows they do this frequently at home, but not very frequently in settings. If we show puzzlement and take an investigatory approach ourselves, showing children that we wonder why too, we can provide this encouragement.

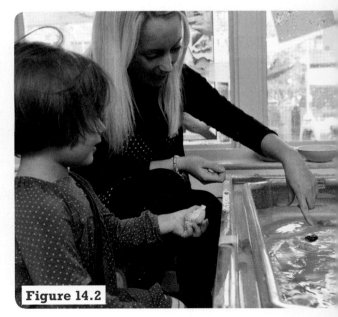

**Figure 14.2**

### Encouraging children to investigate and ask questions

With a group of children in your setting, plan a mini beast hunt in your outdoor area. Ask the children what equipment they think will be helpful, showing them a range of possible equipment, such as transparent boxes and magnifying glasses, as necessary. Talk to the children about what they find and note down some of the things they say. Take photographs so that you can use these to make a display or, even better, a booklet about the investigation.

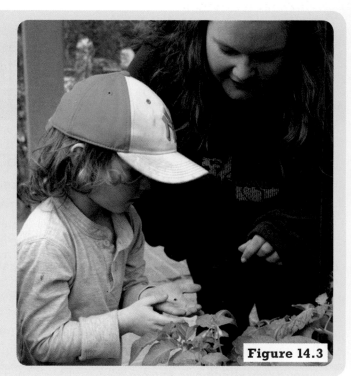

Figure 14.3

## Technology

The final aspect of Understanding the world is technology, but this does not mean sitting in front of a computer, playing games. We need to think of technology in the broadest possible sense, including all the forms of technology that children are likely to encounter in their everyday lives, from the low-tech, such as simple cooking equipment (egg timers, lemon squeezers, egg whisks), to the high-tech of electronic ICT devices.

### Thinking about technology and the provision in your setting

How many different kinds of low-tech devices do children have access to in your setting? Include different types of cooking equipment, such as whisks and lemon squeezers, as well as hole punchers, staplers, water wheels, torches and wheel toys. Think of some open-ended questions to get children interested in looking into how they work.

## High-tech devices

We also need to ensure that children have access to a wide range of high-tech devices, in addition to computers, such as programmable toys, cameras and tape recorders. Children need to develop an awareness of electronic devices in the wider world too, for example, traffic lights and pelican crossings, or electronic gates at train stations or sports centres. Incorporating telephone equipment and computers into role play provides children with opportunities to play with these as they take on a role.

## Guiding principles for choosing software and educational electronic toys

The following set of principles comes from a European-wide research project called DATEC (Developmentally Appropriate Technology in Early Childhood), which began in 1999 and is designed to support early years practitioners in their decision making about what software and educational electronic toys to provide to support young children's use of technology. The seven principles are:

1  Ensure an educational purpose
2  Encourage children to work together and collaborate
3  Integrate with other aspects of curriculum
4  Ensure the child is in control *(open-ended tasks are the best and the child not the adult is in control, with adult support as necessary)*
5  Choose applications that are transparent *(each function should be clearly defined, so for example an action produces an outcome)*
6  Avoid applications containing violence or stereotyping
7  Be aware of health and safety issues *(such as children not sitting for too long at a computer).*

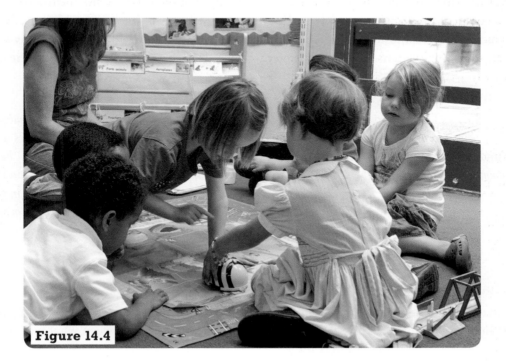

**Figure 14.4**

## Looking at children:
## What do we see?

### Daisy, age 2 years

Daisy has been shown maps from an early age, as there is a map of the world on the kitchen wall at home and a globe that is often used to locate places that are significant to the family – where relations and friends live or visit. She can now locate some countries that are important to her on both the map and the globe. She and her family often travel to visit extended family, none of whom live near her, and her grandmother lives on an island off the north coast of Scotland. Before a long car journey the length of the British Isles, Daisy's father showed her the map of Britain, showing her where she was going and the routes they were to take. Two weeks later, on a short journey in the car, looking at a different map, she said to herself: "Need to go further up there ... and further down, down there," moving her finger up and down as she said the words.

On a walk a few days later, Daisy could identify the difference on a sign between a small map and small drawings. Maps are very much part of her imaginative play too. Playing in a pretend car made by her grandmother out of a crate, a cardboard box, a steering wheel and a stick for a gear lever, the most important thing for Daisy was the map. She put it in the pretend boot and took it out time after time, as she chatted about where she was going. Daisy's interest in and knowledge about maps is one aspect of Understanding the world.

### What we have found out?

This may seem very remarkable for a child of just 2 years, but what is important to the family is most likely to be picked up quickly by the child. Practitioners need to be aware of the knowledge, skills and understanding children bring with them when they attend a setting. An activity such as the one at the beginning of this chapter will help Daisy to build on her sense of the world.

### Zeinaddine, age 3 years 6 months

Zeinaddine's key person wrote: *"Zeinaddine has been watching the caterpillars and chrysalises in the nursery classroom with interest. On a walk in the nursery school garden we found some leaves with holes in and I asked him what he thought had been eating them. 'The Very Hungry Caterpillar,' he replied, remembering the storybook. I encouraged him to look under the plants and in the nooks and crannies of the garden. We found ants, empty snail shells and spiders' webs. Zein's interest turned to the fish in the pond. 'That big one's so big it's going to eat me! It's going to bite me!' We looked closely at the colours of the fish and their tails, fins, gills and eyes. 'He's looking at me. It's a shark!' Zein said. Next we looked at a book about various fish and sharks."*

### What we have found out?

Zeinaddine is showing deep interest in what he sees. His awareness of a range of living things is developing, supported by his key person. He makes connections between what he knows from storybooks and what he sees in real life.

## What the experts say
Forest Schools: Extending children's understanding of nature and the environment

A Forest School is usually an area of natural woodland or natural environment that is being used to provide an educational experience for young children, usually from 2 years upwards. It might be an area within the setting's grounds, a nearby school's grounds or may involve a trip in a minibus to a woodland area. Many Forest Schools are used by older children too. Forest Schools first began in England in the 1990s, taking ideas from ongoing work in Scandinavian countries where it began in the 1950s. It has grown significantly in recent years in Britain.

The aim of the Forest School is to provide children with experiences of the natural world (within strict safety routines) that they would not otherwise have. This is particularly important for children from more built-up areas, giving them opportunities to explore using all their senses, develop their thinking and creative skills as well as using their physical skills. At least one member of staff needs to be trained as a Forest School leader and others are trained in how to support the children. The training ensures practitioners understand not only how to run a Forest School to ensure it is safe and secure, but about how adults can support and guide children's learning. For more information, see the Useful websites section at the end of this chapter.

## Effective practice:
What do we need to do?

Much of the effective practice described in other chapters in this book also applies to supporting children's understanding of the world. For *People and communities*, it means providing children with a breadth of experience as they grow from toddlers into 3- and 4-year-olds, so that they see themselves as belonging to the wider community. For *The world*, first-hand experiences are essential, but also taking an enquiry-based approach, encouraging children to be curious and questioning. For *Technology*, first-hand experiences are vital.

- Provide plenty of books and stories to support children's learning in all aspects of Understanding the world. Stories that accurately and positively depict people in cultural settings other than British set a good model.
- Take children on outings in the local community and further afield to visit environments that are different from where they live. Invite family members to come along. Make sure the safety rules for outings in your setting are adhered to.
- Involve families in the activities you plan, perhaps in helping you find recipes or becoming involved in a cooking activity, or talking about their work or home life.

## People and communities

- Ensure every child feels that they are an important member of the group. Find out about children's favourite songs they sing at home, favourite toys, activities and events at home, and find ways for the children to share these with the other children in your setting.
- Help children understand and celebrate similarities and differences between people, for example using Persona Dolls as well as books and stories. (For more information about Persona Dolls see Chapters 2 and 4.)

## The world

- Encourage children's curiosity by taking an enquiry-based approach, so that children feel at ease to explore and find out about things that interest them. Help them too to develop interest in things they have not previously shown interest in.
- Provide plenty of opportunities to explore the world outdoors, from babies upwards. Talk with them about what they are experiencing. Introduce new (and correct) vocabulary such as the names of mini beasts. Take photographs and make books with them about their investigations.

## Technology

- Provide a breadth of safe, low-technology tools, making sure, once children have had some time to explore for themselves, that you draw their attention to how things work. For low technology, this could be through a planned activity experimenting with different types of whisks, lemon squeezers or tweezers, and other devices for picking things up, for example.
- Provide a breadth of appropriate high technology, for 3- to 5-year-olds, making sure you address the DATEC principles highlighted earlier in this chapter.

## Case study: Understanding children's understanding of the world

At Woodlands Park, staff working with the over-3s often use projects to develop their support for children's learning. This is how the photography project came about. Working with an artist who often supports the setting, they set up the project to:

- teach the children about photography and how to use cameras (cameras are very much a part of their lives)
- enable them to express themselves through their own photographs and talk about these
- develop a project together with the children's families.

The project had a significant impact on children's learning in all three aspects of Understanding the world: People and communities, The world, and Technology. First, the children learnt how to use the cameras, taking their own photographs of things that interested them in the nursery environment. These were shared with the parents, giving the parents a view of the setting from their child's perspective. The next step was an outing with the children, cameras and parents to the local park. On the way the children photographed what interested them. The photographs tell a very different story from the one that would have resulted from the adults taking the photos. The children photographed the leaves on the ground, the trunk of a tall tree, the road, a bench, the local cafe, the wheels of a car and several snaps of a cat snoozing on a dustbin.

The photographs were printed off and laminated. Now another outing was arranged to display the photos exactly where the children took them, for example, hung on a tree or a fence or tied to a hedge. This really got the local community wondering: "How did these photographs suddenly appear?" and "Why were these objects photographed?" were comments heard frequently in the streets and in the park!

## Chapter summary

This chapter will have helped you:
- understand what this important area of learning, Understanding the world, means and what it covers
- reflect on what your setting is already providing to support children's learning and what further experiences and activities can be provided.

## Further reading and references

Cole, J. and Davy, A. (2009) 'The Sky is the Limit', supplementary leaflet, *The Sky is the Limit*, Early Education, London

Evangelou, M., Sylva, K., Kyriacou, M., Wild, M. and Glenny, G. (2009) 'Early Years Learning and Development: Literature Review', DCSF Research Report RR176. Available to download from: www.education.gov.uk/publications/RSG/publicationDetail/Page1/DCSF-RR176

Garrick, R. (2006) *Minibeasts and More: Young Children Investigating the Natural World*, Early Education, London

Siraj-Blatchford, I. and Siraj-Blatchford J. (2003) *More Than Computers: Information and Communication Technology in the Early Years*, Early Education, London

### Useful websites

DATEC guidance on the seven principles of using technology in the early years: www.datec.org.uk/guidance/DATEC7.pdf

Forest Schools: www.forestschools.com

## Chapter 15

# Expressive arts and design

## In this chapter we will be looking at:

➤ what this EYFS specific area of learning, Expressive arts and design, covers

➤ some observations of children exploring aspects of this area of learning

➤ what an expert has to tell us about how we can support children's learning in Expressive arts and design

➤ some examples of what you can do to ensure your practice is effective in Expressive arts and design.

## Introduction

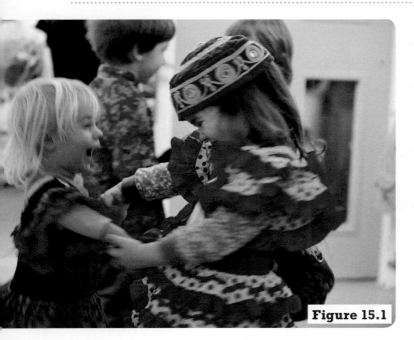

**Figure 15.1**

Expressive arts and design takes countless forms in the early years. In this photograph, for example, we see some 2- and 3-year-olds dancing. The two girls love dressing up, and every day they put on flouncy dresses, with hats and bags as important accessories. This afternoon, having dressed up, they begin to dance, spinning round and round joyfully. Two boys watch this creative play developing. They run to the home corner and find two boys' jackets, put them on and join the dancers. You can see them dancing just behind the girls. They are expressing their delight through dancing.

## The EYFS specific area of learning, Expressive arts and design, tells us:

"Expressive arts and design involves enabling children to explore and play with a wide range of media and materials, as well as providing opportunities and encouragement for sharing their thoughts, ideas and feelings through a variety of activities in art, music, movement, dance, role-play, and design and technology."

(EYFS Statutory Framework, 2012)

This area of learning was previously called Creative development, although what this area covers has not changed. The reason for the change of name to Expressive arts and design was to focus "attention more clearly on children's experiences of exploring and learning about creative and artistic expression" (Tickell, 2011). It is a specific area of learning and, like the other specific areas, links closely to the prime areas of learning. It also links closely to the Characteristics of learning (see Section 2), where *how* children learn is considered, in particular, Playing and exploring and Creating and thinking critically.

## What is this specific area of learning about?

In Expressive arts and design two aspects are highlighted:
- **Exploring and using media and materials**
- **Being imaginative.**

Both aspects cover the many fields of artistic creativeness: art (painting, drawing, making models), music, dance, imaginative play and role play. As they explore an array of artistic experiences, young children engage in creative expression, and the two aspects, exploring and using media and materials and being imaginative, are closely linked. We want children to be imaginative as they explore and use materials, and they cannot be creative without imagination.

For babies and toddlers the creative process is very much an exploratory one, for example exploring the pattern that can be made as they move their hands through spilled yoghurt. Later, as they grow and develop, they will begin to want to represent their own experiences and their imagination, and begin to express their creativity in many different ways. Loris Malaguzzi, the inspirational founder of the Reggio Emilia Preschools in Italy, calls this creative expression "the Hundred Languages of Children". This is how he put it:

*"The child*
*is made of one hundred.*
*The child has*
*A hundred languages*
*A hundred hands*
*A hundred thoughts*
*A hundred ways of thinking*
*Of playing, of speaking.*
*A hundred always a hundred*

*Ways of listening of marvelling of loving*
*A hundred joys*
*For singing and understanding*
*A hundred worlds*
*To discover*
*A hundred worlds*
*To invent*
*A hundred worlds*
*To dream"* *(Malaguzzi, 1993)*

# Exploring and using media and materials

## Making marks: drawing and painting

Babies begin to explore mark-making very young, perhaps when they are first able to sit up independently, using their hands and fingers in any materials where marks can be made. Exploring mark-making continues into adulthood and we need to encourage it if we are to support children to express themselves creatively. Media such as cornflour, wet clay or paint are great for children to explore the marks they can make on the type of large scale necessary for their developing fine motor skills. Mark-making on a smaller scale, using smaller paper for example, should only be introduced when children's fine motor skills are mature enough for them to handle tools such as brushes, chalks, crayons and pens. Using their hands to make marks should continue, as this is the most direct mark-making tool.

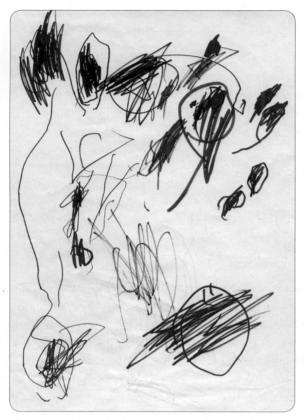

**Figure 15.2** Daisy's mark-making. Notice how Daisy, age 2 years, has made lines as well enclosing spaces deliberately and infilled the enclosed space

It is important that practitioners and parents do not expect certain kinds of marks or drawings, and ensure children have the freedom to explore their mark-making for themselves. Even when children begin to label their drawings and paintings as representations of things and people, their marks will not conform to our adult ideas of representations and we should not expect them to. We need to encourage them to make marks for the pleasure of it; sometimes (but usually not before the age of 2 to 3 years) this will be a representation, but sometimes it will be an exploration of what is possible. Showing interest in what they are doing and celebrating achievements is the best form of encouragement.

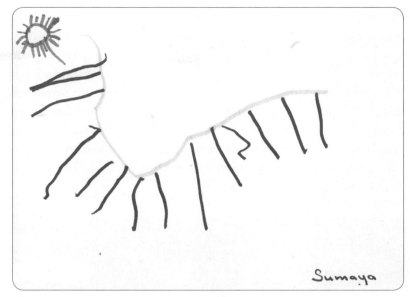

**Figure 15.3** Sumaya, age 3 years 8 months, has drawn a caterpillar and the sun. Her school had recently hatched caterpillars from eggs. There is a real sense of caterpillar movement in her drawing

## 3D modelling

As babies and young children explore the properties of shapes they also begin creating things in three dimensions. Wooden blocks for building and construction are ideal, as they are open-ended and can be used in so many different shapes. Construction sets are often less creative as they need to be clicked together in specific ways. Modelling with recycled materials provides children with a wealth of different shapes to explore, firing the imagination in new ways. Modelling with media such as clay is essential too.

## Activity

### The creative workshop

*For 2- to 5-year-olds:*

1 Does your setting have a creative workshop where children help themselves to the tools and resources they need? If so, how well organised is it? Are the resources visibly arranged on open shelves so that children can easily find the resources they need?

2 Do you have a good supply of different types of resources (boxes of all shapes and sizes, lolly sticks and matchsticks, cardboard tubes, bottle tops, paper, ribbon, fabric)?

3 Is there a good supply of different joining materials – tape, glue, string, rubber bands? Do the children know how to use these?

4 If your setting does not have an area like this, how can you create one?

*For under-2s:*

The same resources as described above, so long as they are safe and clean, can be provided but without the joining materials.

## Music

Babies tune in to the musicality of the voices around them very early in their lives. Soon we see them moving their bodies delightedly to the rhythm of music, and copying you clapping to the rhythm. Singing rhymes and songs and giving young children opportunities to regularly explore a range of instruments and things that make sounds is important. With encouragement and support children will begin to be able to use a percussion instrument to copy a beat, repeat a beat and make up a pattern of beats. They need experience of listening to a wide range of different music, with different tempo, volume, pitch and instruments, not as background music, which does not help them tune their ears in to the sounds, but at times when they can listen more attentively.

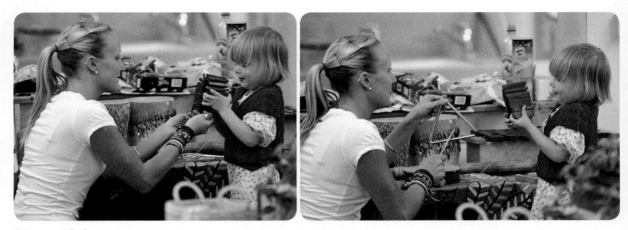

**Figure 15.4** This child is being shown how to use an unfamiliar percussion instrument – she quickly learns how to use it

## Activity

### A percussion corner

Create a space for exploring sound outdoors. A washing line tied across an underused corner can be ideal. Hang a range of everyday items on the line that will make different sounds, for example an old saucepan, a frying pan and a large tin can or an old kettle, different-size pieces of wood, a thick cardboard tube, a plastic bottle with some dry sand or gravel in it. Provide sticks or beaters for children to hit the sound-makers with (these can be tied to the line too). Encourage children to listen to the sounds they hear.

## Movement and dance

When we think of listening to music with young children, we often think of movement and dance too. It is important that children are encouraged to try out different movements, swaying and spinning, and to let movement flow to the music as well as using movements that contrast, such as slow and fast.

## Exploring or teaching children skills?

Young children need as many opportunities as possible to explore a wide variety of experiences of media and materials, presented in inviting ways to tempt the children to get involved. But there are also techniques and processes that children will need to be taught. Different types of artistic experiences (art, dance, music) require different skills and techniques. Choosing the right time to introduce the technique comes from observing the child, knowing that they are ready for it, while they are showing interest. Exploration comes first.

# Being imaginative

There has already been considerable coverage in this book about children being imaginative and most of the observations of children in each chapter show children using their imaginations as they play, think and do. Pretend play, role play and fantasy play are key ways in which children explore the world using their imagination. Practitioners and parents need to encourage children to be imaginative. Help to let their imaginations flow, giving them time to think and by providing thought-provoking things to interest them.

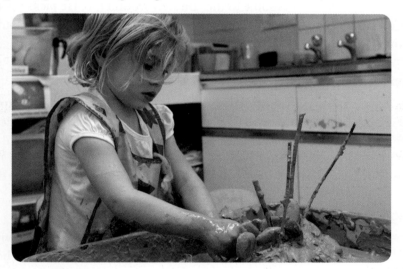

**Figure 15.5** This child is deeply involved in creating a castle with wet clay. She spent a considerable amount of the afternoon creating this

## Activity

Look at the observation of Almas on the next page. Allowing children to explore creative materials in flexible ways can be messy, but it is important to let children's explorations flow.

1 How is this type of exploration encouraged in your setting, and how often?

2 If this was your setting, what would you do to ensure that cleaning and tidying up were part of an enjoyable and creative experience for Almas and her peers?

3 List what you would do to ensure tidying up and cleaning remain an enjoyable part of the whole creative experience. Include the tools and resources you might use and think about how long you would need.

4 Think about what your role in supporting the children would be.

## Looking at children:
## What do we see?

### William, age 19 months

William explores the resources in the graphics area: chalks, coloured pencils, and so on. He makes some lines on paper and on a sticky note. He sticks the note onto his mark-making, saying "Yeah!" excitedly. He moves to the easel and makes marks on the paper, first using a brush, then his fingers and hands, making delighted sounds as he does so. He uses his hands to make prints on the paper, then tries with some shapes he finds on a nearby table. He offers paintbrushes to other children, then paints his key person's hands with the brush, laughing as he does so, then goes off to wash his own hands by himself.

Another observation, taken on the same day, shows William exploring the home corner. He puts some soft toys and then a doll on the chairs next to him and begins feeding them with the available plastic food. He offers some to the children around too. He picks up a dressing-up hat and puts it on his head and goes to the cooker. He returns to the doll and puts it in the doll's house, saying, "Sleep baby!" and covering it with a blanket.

### What have we found out?

In the first observation we see William developing an interest in and exploring the tools for graphics, and just beginning to make marks. In the second observation he is playing imaginatively. We have seen William's interest in role play in other observations in this book. He happily plays alongside others, many of whom are older. Although he is not yet playing a role, he is already, at 19 months, pretending, feeding the toys and putting the doll to bed.

### Almas, age 2 years 4 months

Paint has been provided for children directly on the table, for them to use with tools, such as sponges and rollers, or with their hands. Almas mixes the paints together with both her hands on the table, then makes marks with her fingers, and as more colours are offered she accepts them. After a while she goes to wash the paints off her hands, then begins to use a roller, including rolling the paint up her arms, then on her face, using one colour for her hands and a different one for her face. She starts to play peek-a-boo, using the rollers and her fingers to cover her eyes and peep out.

### What have we found out?

Almas is thoroughly enjoying her experience with paint and the activity is on a large scale, with flexibility for children to explore with their hands or with tools. Almas is well organised, exploring and experimenting with the paint on her body and using tools. She turns this experience into an imaginative game.

## What the experts say
## Cultivating creativity

Tina Bruce is well known for her work in supporting early years practitioners to enhance children's creative development. Her books contain many examples of children developing and using their creativity and imagination as they develop their thinking and learning. They also contain detailed explanations of the role of the practitioner (and parent) in providing the type of support that children need. In her book, *Cultivating Creativity in Babies, Toddlers and Young Children* (Bruce, 2011), she specifically addresses the aspects of Expressive arts and design, as well as helping the reader to understand the importance of creativity in all learning.

She points out that children's life experiences are vital to creativity. "Creativity does not come from nowhere. It feeds off our experiences. It depends on them for creative ideas to develop" (Bruce, 2011). Looking at research on the creative process, Bruce notes how it starts with the idea of "incubation". Although "After incubation, a creation might be hatched out", she emphasises that most creative ideas do *not* end in a "creation" (a product). This is particularly true of young children, where most of the child's interest is usually on the process. She also talks about "Giving children the technical know-how". As she says: "Every subject has its technical know-how", and she follows this up with an important point: "Remember that you need to help the child make a basic technique fit them as an individual. They need to use the basics to suit them as a unique person" (Bruce, 2011).

## Effective practice:
## What do we need to do?

Effective practice in Expressive arts and design means ensuring, from babies onwards, that children are provided with a breadth of experiences, inside and outside, to explore and "feed creative ideas" (Bruce, 2011). The arts for children are about exploring creative processes and developing their own creative expressions. Giving children templates to draw around or pictures to colour in is *not* recommended in any circumstances. Neither is every child producing the same product for a festival or any other reason. This is not creative expression, does not support the child's creativity and is likely to damage their confidence in making their own creations.

- Make time to talk with parents about children's creative experiences at home and at your setting. Research by Anning and Ring (2004) looked at the differences between children's drawings at home and in settings. They noted that the home was generally a better environment for children to express themselves through drawing than in their settings, as parents tended to be better tuned in to their child's creative ideas and mark-making. We need to make sure that in our settings children are given the time they need with adults who tune in to them.

- Think about the different aspects of your role in promoting and providing opportunities for children's expressive arts and design, by:
  - being there for the child, observing what the child is doing and being available to support through talking with the child about the processes they are using (not "What is it?" but "I like the way you are adding the yellow" or "I like the way you are making that sound by tapping your fingers lightly on the drum").
  - finding new or different resources to support particular interests or spark off new ideas
  - supporting children to develop technical know-how when children are not busy in the exploratory stage, by showing them the particular techniques appropriate to the experience they are involved in – for example, teaching a child how to remove the excess water from a paintbrush when using palette paints, how to use scissors, a tape dispenser or a hole puncher.

## Activity

### Observing a child exploring materials and media

Choose a child to observe while they are engaged in different creative experiences, for example mark-making (painting, drawing), using blocks and construction (3D) and playing physically outdoors. Does there appear to be a theme to the marks they make that can also be seen in the construction play and physical play? You may be seeing the child's repeating patterns of behaviour (schema); they may be using straight lines or be interested in rotational movement or in covering things up. Knowing this can help you plan further experiences. To find out more about schemas, see the Further reading and references section at the end of this chapter.

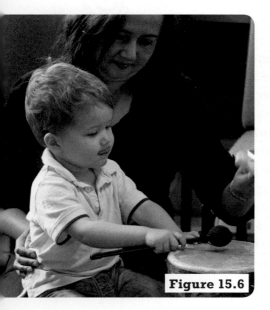

**Figure 15.6**

## Exploring and using media and materials

- Make sure the learning environment is rich in potential for creative and artistic expression, in music, dance, drama, role play and art. Remember that the world outdoors lends itself to inspiration from the weather and the sights, sounds and textures of the environment.
- Set up a well-resourced creative workshop area. Resources and tools need to be well cared for, so involve children in taking responsibility and caring for them.
- Provide musical instruments for babies and children to explore and try out, as well as providing times when these can be used in small groups, along with singing.
- Sing songs frequently and encourage children to sing as they play.
- Provide a range of music from different cultures for children to listen to, with different rhythms and tempo.

## Being imaginative

- Read, talk about and, if appropriate, act out stories that will fire the children's imagination.
- Provide plenty of time and space for creative processes so that children can incubate their ideas and try out their own creative techniques.

---

### Case study: Exploring and using materials and media – clay

At Woodlands Park, exploring clay – a wonderful material for children's exploration and creative expression – has been a particular focus of attention for staff development and supporting children's all-round learning. Working with an artist who supported them in the initial stages, the project has gone from strength to strength. The aim was for children to explore and experiment with the clay using all their senses. It became a great opportunity for conversation with the children about what it feels like and what you can do with it. As Cath, the artist, said: "At first they become familiar with the clay presented in different ways, such as in a large lump or rolled flat, on its own. Later, natural materials such as wire, buttons, lolly and match sticks are introduced."

As the children explore they are not only developing their creative ideas, understanding of the material itself and language, but also their mathematical understanding (weight, shape and space). Cath and the staff ran a very successful workshop for parents about the work they were doing with clay, making the children's interests and ideas visible to the parents and giving parents and children an opportunity to explore together.

*(With thanks to Cath Rive)*

---

### Chapter summary

This chapter will have helped you:
- ➤ understand more about this specific area of learning
- ➤ reflect on what you can do to support children to express themselves creatively and develop their imaginations through art, music, dance and role play.

## Further reading and references

Anning, A. and Ring, K. (2004) *Making Sense of Children's Drawings*, Open University Press/McGraw-Hill, London

Bruce, T. (2009) *Early Childhood: A Guide for Students*, Sage Publications, London

Bruce, T. (2011) *Cultivating Creativity: For Babies, Toddlers and Young Children* (2nd edn.), Hodder Education, London

Bruce, T., Meggitt, C. and Grenier, J. (2010) *Childcare and Education*, Hodder Education, London

Cole, J. and Davy, A. (2009) 'The Sky is the Limit', supplementary leaflet, *The Sky is the Limit*, Early Education, London

Featherstone, S., Louis, S. and Beswick, C. (2008) *Again, Again!: Understanding Schemas in Young Children*, Featherstone Education Ltd, London

Malaguzzi, L. (1993) 'No way. The hundred is there' in: *The Hundred Languages of Children: The Reggio Emilia Approach to Early Childhood Education*, Edwards, C., Gandini, L. and Forman, G. (eds.), Ablex Publishing Corporation, Norwood, NJ

Ouvry, M. (2004) *Sounds like Playing: Music and the Early Years Curriculum*, Early Education, London

Ring, K. (2010) 'Drawing and Writing Outdoors: Prioritising Playfulness', supplementary leaflet, *The Sky is the Limit*, Early Education, London

## Useful websites

Education Scotland, Early Years, Nine features of the key principles: Play: www.ltscotland.org.uk/earlyyears/prebirthtothree/nationalguidance/ninefeatures/play.asp

# Section 5: Assessment in the EYFS

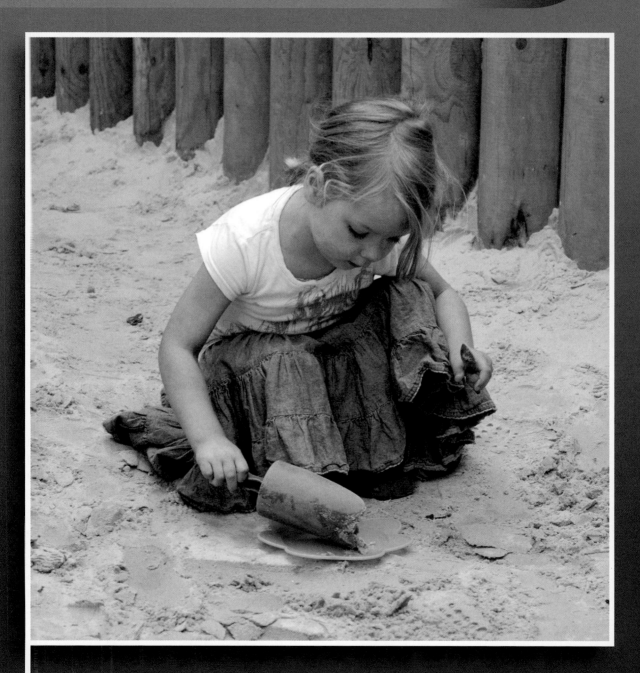

The final section of the book comprises just one very important chapter:

Chapter 16 Assessing children's learning.

# Assessing children's learning

## In this chapter we will be looking at:

➤ why, what and how to assess children's learning and the observation, assessment and planning cycle

➤ how to summarise children's achievements, including the summary for the statutory **'Progress check at age 2'** and the summative assessment before a child moves to a reception class

➤ the work of some experts who have been influential in helping practitioners to develop their assessment processes

➤ how to ensure practice is effective, with some examples from settings developing their assessment processes.

## Introduction

There are two processes of assessment that we will be looking at in this chapter: the ongoing *formative assessment*, which we will look at first, and summarising children's achievements, including the *summative assessments* that practitioners are asked to complete at certain times.

The early years settings featured in this book constantly reflect on their observation, assessment and planning processes, to ensure they are doing the very best for all the children. Three of these settings have recently decided to adopt the Learning Story approach, which you will find out more about in this chapter. They feel this way of assessing the children's learning works so well because it naturally involves the children and parents in the assessment process. The practitioners not only find Learning Stories a very manageable way to assess children, they also love doing them!

Denise, a senior teacher and acting deputy in one Children's Centre, said: "All the children and parents like the Learning Stories. Each key person puts them in the child's profile (record) with the child." It is an ideal time to sit together, look at the photographs and talk about the child's achievements. Karen and Jess, in another Children's Centre, said: "Assessment *mustn't* be a burden! Since using Learning Stories we have found that all the staff are enthusiastic about doing them." Read on to find out more about the processes they are using and how they meet the requirements of the revised EYFS in the process.

# The EYFS requirements on ongoing formative assessment tell us:

*"Assessment plays an important part in helping parents, carers and practitioners to recognise children's progress, understand their needs, and to plan activities and support."*

(EYFS Statutory Framework, 2012)

Practitioners use ongoing or formative assessment in their day-to-day work with children. Much of it is *informal* and involves the thinking process you go through as you respond to what you see the children do, or hear what they communicate to you, moment by moment. This means being observant and listening well as you interact with the children. Only some of this is written down or photographed by practitioners. In Chapter 3, the EYFS 2008 commitment, Observation, assessment and planning, was discussed. In 2012 the revised version made no changes to the requirements about ongoing assessment. The wording has changed slightly, but the requirements remain the same, with an emphasis on the importance of observing children as the basis of assessment.

*"Ongoing assessment (also known as formative assessment), is an integral part of the learning and development process. It involves practitioners observing children to understand their level of achievement, interests and learning styles, and then to shape learning experiences for each child reflecting those observations. In their interactions with children, practitioners should respond to their own day-to-day observations about children's progress, and observations that parents and carers share."*

(EYFS Statutory Framework, 2012)

This ongoing assessment leads to the summative assessments that practitioners take at certain points, some of which are requirements, such as the Progress check for parents when their child is 2 years, and the Early Years Foundation Stage Profile at the end of the reception year.

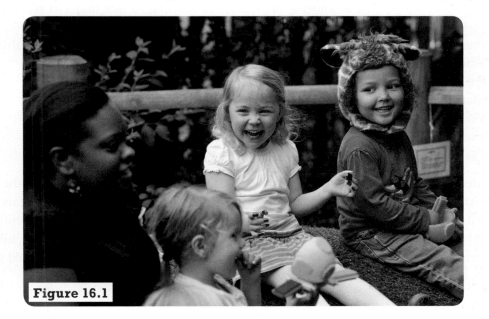

**Figure 16.1**

# What is this theme about?

## Ongoing formative assessment in the EYFS

### Why do we need to observe and assess children?

The main reason we need to assess children's learning and development is so that we can plan appropriately for them and ensure that children are making progress in their learning and development. As the EYFS in 2008, quoted in Chapter 3, says: "All planning starts with observing children in order to understand and consider their current interests, development and learning" (EYFS, 2008). Unless we regularly observe children we will not know if our provision for them is right or what to do next to extend this. The richest source of information about their learning will come from observations of children at play and in self-chosen activities.

The second reason for observing and making assessments is to share with parents what we are finding out about their children. We need to *involve* the parents too, as they know their children best, and what they see their children do at home is important. Putting together the evidence from parents with the evidence from practitioners in the setting, we are able to develop a fully rounded assessment, showing the child's achievements holistically. This helps us to get the planning right.

Often other professionals, such as health care professionals, need to be involved in supporting the children to develop and learn. Practitioners' observations and assessments have a vital role in helping, side by side with parents, to inform other professionals about the child.

### What to assess

On the training courses I run on assessment in the early years, I always ask practitioners what they feel they really need to know about children's learning so that they can plan effectively. The answers are invariably:

- What interests and motivates the child or baby most? What are their likes and dislikes?
- What do the children get really enthusiastic about?
- How do they approach play or any particular task?
- What seems to make them feel most confident?
- How are they relating to others?
- How are they communicating?
- How are their physical skills developing?

This demonstrates that practitioners find the most useful information is both how the children are learning and how they are progressing in the prime areas of learning. It seems that the revised EYFS has got it just right to prioritise the characteristics of learning (see Section 2) and the prime areas of learning (see Section 3)! This does *not* mean we ignore how children are learning and developing in the specific areas of learning (Section 4), as we also need to ensure we are supporting them effectively in these too.

## Activity

### What to assess

Find out about what the other practitioners you work with think is most important to know about children's learning. If your setting has a policy about assessment, or the written information given to parents includes information about assessment, how does what the practitioners told you match up with the policy? If you are a student, share your findings with your mentor/supervisor.

### How to assess

In Chapter 3, the 'Observation–Assessment–Planning' cycle was referred to. The diagram below shows the cycle, which begins with practitioners observing children and talking with the children's parents. The following pages explain the processes within this cycle in more detail.

### The observation, assessment and planning cycle

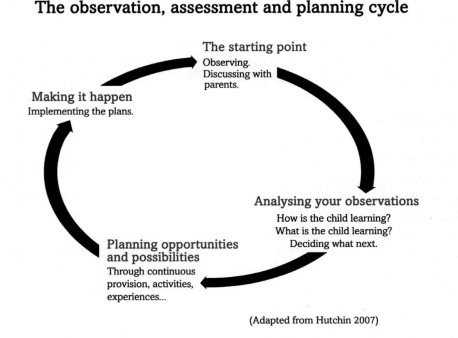

The starting point
Observing.
Discussing with
parents.

Making it happen
Implementing the plans.

Analysing your observations
How is the child learning?
What is the child learning?
Deciding what next.

Planning opportunities
and possibilities
Through continuous
provision, activities,
experiences...

(Adapted from Hutchin 2007)

**Figure 16.2** The 'Observation–Assessment–Planning' cycle (adapted from Hutchin, 2007)

# Observing

This is the first part of the cycle. You will find lots of advice about how best to observe and assess in books for early childhood students and practitioners, but any method you use must show what children *can* do, valuing the child's achievements. It must be fit for purpose (to plan the most appropriate learning experiences and opportunities for the children) and manageable. The Tickell Review in 2011 expressed concern that too much time was being spent on "the paperwork associated with ongoing assessment", and not enough time was being spent on interacting with them. This is reiterated in the EYFS Statutory Framework: "Assessment should not entail prolonged breaks from interaction with children, nor require excessive paperwork." To address this issue, I recommend that to gain a comprehensive picture of the child's achievements a mix of methods of observing is needed, as set out below. The method you choose depends on what you are doing at the time.

## Participant observations

For most of the time practitioners should be involved in interacting with the children, in their play and self-chosen activities and in planned activities. As you interact with the children, jot down notes of anything you see the children do that is *different and new*, and that you have not already noted before. Remember that if it does not seem *significant*, there is no need to write it down. Most settings use self-adhesive labels or sticky notes for this, which can then easily be stuck into the child's record.

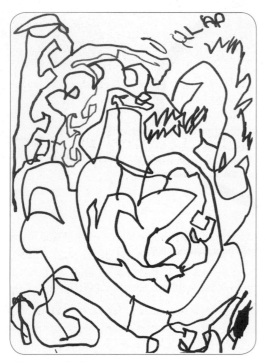

**Figure 16.3** Zein's drawing: a drawing which is new and different from before

## Catch-as-you-can notes

Sometimes you will see something happening in passing that you were not involved in. If this is something *new and different* from what you already know, and seems significant, jot it down.

For both these kinds of observations, you do not need to include every possible detail, unless you have been asked by a specialist professional to do so, for example.

## Photographs, video and mark-making

Digital cameras are a wonderful asset to observations, enabling you to capture the learning as it happens and to share it with parents and the children. For tips on using digital cameras for observations, see the Helpful tip on page 34 of Chapter 3.

## Conversations with the child

A conversation with a child (this can be a non-verbal, gestured conversation) can be well worth noting down, because the conversation can indicate a child's interests, growing vocabulary and general language development.

## Observations, samples and photographs from home

Parents have a greater role in children's learning and development than anyone else in their lives, so inviting parents to bring photographs of what the child is doing at home, samples of their drawings or things they are making and their own observations makes very good sense indeed. In fact, the EYFS Profile, the statutory assessment of children at the end of the EYFS, is the *only* statutory assessment in which information gathered from parents about their child's learning and development at home can be and should be included (see Chapter 5).

## Occasional focused observations

Although the types of observations mentioned above will give you lots of snippets of information about how and what children are learning and developing, it is likely to present a bit of a patchwork and you may have much more information about some children than others. The occasional longer, focused observation, where the observer stands back to watch for a few minutes to observe the child in play or a self-chosen activity, can be *invaluable* because you can find out so much. Vygotsky tells us that in play children are operating at their highest level, so we must make sure we capture this (see Chapter 4).

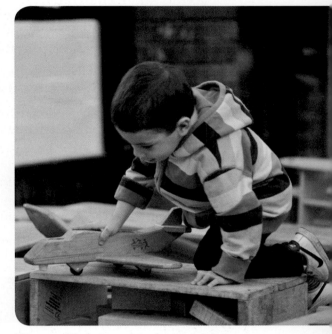

**Figure 16.4** Observing children at play is invaluable

Three to four minutes of observing is usually ample time, but you may also want to come back and look again later. A few minutes of thinking time after you have made your observation is important too. Photographs come into their own in these types of observations, greatly reducing the need for copious note taking. Effective settings and schools try to ensure there is one of these standing-back observations per child every three months, sometimes more frequently if the children are younger or if there is a concern about a child's development.

## From observing to assessing

Observations need thinking about and analysing. In every chapter of this book in the Looking at children sections, there are observations of two children and each is followed by a section called What have we found out? This is the analysis – the assessment part of the cycle in Figure 16.2. We need to ask ourselves: what are we finding out about *what* the child is learning? What is the child showing interest in and how? What skills are being developed? Think about the characteristics of learning: *how* is the child learning?

## Time to reflect

### The characteristics of learning: How are children learning?

The following points will be helpful when analysing observations of children, looking for evidence of how the child is learning.

### Playing and exploring

Is there evidence of the child:

➤ finding out and exploring, e.g. showing curiosity and particular interests?

➤ playing with what they know, e.g. pretending, representing their experiences in their play, taking on a role and acting out experiences?

➤ being willing to have a go, e.g. initiating an activity, trying something out, taking risks and challenging her/himself?

### Active learning

Is there evidence of the child:

➤ being involved and concentrating?

➤ enjoying achieving what they set out to do, e.g. enjoying the challenge and feeling pleased with their achievements?

➤ keeping on trying, showing persistence?

### Creating and thinking critically

Is there evidence of the child:

➤ having their own ideas and thinking up their own ways of solving problems?

➤ making connections, e.g. using what they know to learn new things, noticing patterns and using these to begin to predict?

➤ choosing ways to do things, e.g. making decisions and planning, sometimes reflecting back too?

## Development Matters

The non-statutory guidance 'Development Matters in the Early Years Foundation Stage' is very helpful in showing what young children's learning may look like in a general way, especially for working out what progress looks like in each area of learning and development. It begins by stating clearly that:

*"Children have a right… to provision which enables them to develop their personalities, talents and abilities irrespective of ethnicity, culture or religion, home language, family background, learning difficulties, disabilities or gender."*

(Development Matters, 2012)

It makes clear links between the four themes and principles of the EYFS (covered in Section 1 in this book) and how and what children learn. The tables begin with the 'Characteristics of effective learning' (covered in Section 2 in this book) – then come the areas of learning and development. There is information about what learning may look like (under A Unique Child), related to overlapping age bands. There is useful guidance on the role of the practitioner under the heading Positive Relationships, and 'What adults could provide' under the heading Enabling Environments.

On every page the following important statement is written:

*"Children develop at their own rates, and in their own ways. The development statements and their order should not be taken as necessary steps for individual children. They should not be used as checklists. The age/stage bands overlap because these are not fixed boundaries but suggest a typical range of development."*

## Using Development Matters

In analysing your observations, the first step is to think about what the observation is showing. Development Matters can be a useful guide, but it is unlikely to match exactly with what you saw in any particular observation, or what you heard a child say. It is particularly useful when writing a summary of a child's achievement and for tracking children's progress and helping you to plan in the longer term. The Characteristics of Effective Learning section is particularly helpful for planning.

### Activity

Spend some time familiarising yourself with Development Matters, which can be found at: www.early-education.org.uk

Pages 6 and 7 provide some information about the Characteristics of effective learning. Compare this with the information provided in the Effective practice sections of Chapters 6, 7 and 8 in this book (pages 91–93, 106–8 and 121–23).

Now look at the sections of the age group you currently work with in each area of learning and development. Make sure you look at both age bands where these overlap with the age of children in your group.

## Learning Stories

A Learning Story is a user-friendly and effective way of recording an observation and analysing it. The idea of a Learning Story comes from Margaret Carr, Professor of Education at Waikato University in New Zealand. It is like the focused observation of play discussed earlier, but because of the way it written, it is much more than this. One Learning Story per child every three months (or term) is probably enough, if there are other notes as well, because it tells you so much about so many different aspects of learning. The great thing about the Learning Story approach is that you are including the parents' and the child's own view too. In Chapter 10 we see Austin's key person sharing his Learning Story with him and how it is helping him to reflect on his own learning. This is just one example of how Learning Stories can be so effective, and this way of working is being used across the age range, from babies upwards.

A Learning Story can be about the learning and development of one child, or it can be a group story about several children playing, exploring and learning together. Learning Stories are usually full of photographs of the event in the story. There is not a right way to write a Learning Story, but it is important that it is about something the child initiated: "what the child or children started to do on their own or how the child or children responded in their own way to an invitation or provocation they have been offered" (Drummond, 2010).

It is called a Learning *Story* because it is written up as a narrative or story about the particular significant episode of play. In this way the observer can write in the first person, "I saw", and the child or children become "you" (for example, "I saw you playing with ..."). The point of doing it this way is that it can be so easily shared with the child and with the parent, and it feels so much more real to everyone as a record of an event. Like a good picture book, the illustrations (in this case mainly photographs) can tell much of the story, but it does need some words as well. You will not be surprised to know that many of the observations in this book come from Learning Stories collected by practitioners in different settings.

The story is then analysed, with a heading such as the one found in every chapter of this book: What have we found out? However, as the story is to be written as a story to the child and family, *What it means* is a better heading for this section, and then it can be written to the child. In Chapter 9 the Learning Story of Tanuj is written in this way. After the analysis (what it means) there is space for the child's view and the parents' views. Once their views are gathered, the possible points for planning are added in the section called Opportunities and possibilities. See the Learning Story of Eilish later in this chapter. In Chapter 8, page 120, the discussion with Malachy's mother was very important in deciding what to plan next.

## From the assessment to planning and making it happen

This is the final stage of the ongoing assessment process and encapsulates the whole purpose of assessment: to be used for planning. Making it easy to manage is important, too, and the link between assessment and planning is often called assessment for learning.

### Linking assessment to day-to-day planning

This is about making your planning flexible enough to make sure you can respond to what is happening. For example, thinking about the Learning Story on Eilish later in this chapter (see pages 226 and 227), her key person may want to ensure that the clay is put out the next day too, even though dough or cornflour may have been planned. She may also want to make sure a story with story props is available. This is an immediate response, to catch the moment and extend Eilish's learning.

### In the longer term: Summarising children's achievements

From time to time the key person needs to reflect on the child's learning and ask how well the child is doing. Is there anything else that needs to be done to support the child, not just looking at one event the child was involved in, but at all the notes in the record, along with other things observed and heard which were not written down? Before making the summary, carry out a focused observation or collect a Learning Story on the child.

This seems to work best in the following way:

1 The key person looks through and summarises everything in the record so far (or since the last summary was made) for one to two children a week.

2 Do this for each child once every three months (or once per term). With younger children you may want to do this more frequently, perhaps once every two months.

3 The key person can do this *with* the child. It is a brilliant opportunity for the child to reflect on their own learning and talk about the photographs and examples of mark-making, and so on. It works with all age groups too. You will see examples of this at the beginning of Chapter 8 and at the end of Chapter 10.

4 As you summarise, take a look at Development Matters. Many settings ask key persons to highlight appropriate statements in Development Matters at this point, to help track the child's progress. First think about the Characteristic of effective learning to decide how the child has been learning. The Positive Relationship and Enabling Environment sections will really help you with planning too.

5 The key person summarises the record. There may be many planning points (Opportunities and Possibilities) already recorded, which need pulling out from the record and listed. It is an ideal opportunity to talk them through, especially with 3- to 5-year-olds. If there are no planning points recorded, now is the time to make them.

6 Make a time to meet with and talk to parents (see the example of William later in this chapter) and ask the parents for their views – about what the child is doing at home and their thoughts on what you have summarised about their child. Then discuss the planning points you are proposing with them.

7 Take these to the next planning meeting. Prioritise the planning points: two to three planning points per child is quite enough.

8 Each key person should follow the same routine.

Now it is time to think in more detail about the planning. Will it be planned through the continuous provision you make for play and children's self-chosen activities? How much adult support will you give? Will it be a focused, adult-led activity?

## Activity

### Summarising children's achievements

Sit down with a child and their record (learning diary, learning journey, profile) – every setting seems to call these something different! Look through it with the child, making time to talk about the parts that the child shows particular interest in. Note down planning points – informally talk to the child about what you think might be a good idea, and ask them for their ideas too. Now look at Development Matters – can you summarise the child's achievements to date by looking at these? Have a look at the Characteristics of effective learning too.

## The Statutory Summative Assessments
## The Progress check at age two
## The EYFS requirement for Summative Assessments tells us:

"When a child is aged between two and three, practitioners must review their progress, and provide parents and/or carers with a short written summary of their child's development in the prime areas. This progress check must identify the child's strengths, and any areas where the child's progress is less than expected. If there are significant emerging concerns, or an identified special educational need or disability, practitioners should develop a targeted plan to support the child's future learning and development involving other professionals."

(EYFS Statutory Framework, 2012)

The progress check is a short written summary, based on the ongoing observational assessment carried out as part of everyday practice, taking account of contributions from parents and, where relevant, other practitioners and professionals involved. If possible, it should be made and shared with parents before the child's 2-year-old Healthy Child check, so that parents can share it with their health visitor.

The intention is that it is written by the child's key person and shared with the parents (usually in draft form), and then finalised – incorporating the discussion with parents. The 'Know How Guide', written by the National Children's Bureau, provides useful guidance and examples of all stages in the process. Keeping track of how the child is progressing, and summarising the records in the way described in this chapter will ensure you are fully prepared for the child's official '2-year-old progress check' for parents. In Chapter 5 in this book, there is useful advice on sharing information with parents.

There is no specific format, and the government have left settings to choose the way that they present the required summary. In the 'Know How Guide', there are 4 examples. In addition to highlighting how the child is progressing in the prime areas of learning, it is always useful to highlight *how* the child is learning. Example 2 in the 'Know How Guide' is particularly useful, as it also incorporates a summary of how the child is learning using the Characteristics of effective learning.

### The EYFS Profile

At the very end of the EYFS phase, when nearly every child is in a reception class in a primary school, the EYFS Profile is to be completed. It is based on the ongoing observations, discussions with parents and conversations with the children carried out throughout the reception year in all seven areas of learning. Teachers are asked to assess children in June of the reception year, when most children are 5 years old or soon will be, against the 17 Early Learning Goal statements and the three Characteristics of effective learning.

## The EYFS requirement for the EYFS Profile tells us:

"In the final term of the year in which the child reaches age five... the EYFS profile must be completed for each child. The profile must reflect: ongoing observation; all relevant records held by the setting; discussions with parents and carers, and any other adults whom the teacher, parents or carer judges can offer a useful contribution."

(EYFS Statutory Framework, 2012)

It goes on to confirm that the *"Year 1 teachers must be given a copy of the Profile, together with a short commentary on each child's skills and abilities in relation to the three Characteristics of effective learning"* to *"assist with the planning of activities in Year 1".*

## Looking at children:
## What do we see?

### A learning story

#### What did you see?

As well as recording significant things you saw, record child's level of involvement and concentration, signs of well-being and the social context – were others involved too? If possible, record what the child said.

*Eilish, today I saw you busily working with the clay. Although you were obviously engaged and enjoying the experience you chatted to me throughout. You started by telling me you were making a boat. "There's water inside and it goes round and round. It's one of those pedally boats." The clay seemed a bit dry for you to work so I suggested you used a little water from the bowl. You did and you continued to mould your clay. "Ben and Holly have a big boat and then a big fish eats it and then they get another one. I saw it on TV," you said. At this point you turned the clay on its side and said: "Then it standed on the edge and started to move backwards!" and you started to laugh.*

#### What learning was in evidence?

*Eilish, you were very involved in using the clay to create objects and you seemed to be using this to tell and retell stories. You used lots of language to describe position as well as develop the story.*

#### Prime areas: PSED, Physical, Communication and language

***PSED***: *You enjoyed chatting to me and seemed very relaxed, enjoying what you were doing.*

***Physical***: *You used your hands well to mould the clay into a boat-like shape.*

***Communication and language***: *You were using lots of language to tell your story and describe position.*

#### Specific areas: Literacy, Maths, UW, Expressive arts/design

***Mathematics***: *You used lots of positional language as you told your story: inside, backwards, and some shape language too: round, edge.*

***Expressive arts/design***: *You created a model of a boat to tell your imaginative story with me – I think this was you retelling a story you had seen on television, but it was your story and creation!*

**Characteristics of learning:** *Anything significant observed?*

**Playing and exploring**: finding out and exploring, using what they know in their play, being willing to have a go

*You were definitely exploring ways to represent your story with clay.*

**Active learning**: being involved and concentrating, keeping on trying, enjoying achieving what they set out to do

*You were very involved, concentrating on your creation and your story, enjoying what you were achieving and persisting with it.*

**Creating and thinking critically**: having their own ideas, using what they know to learn new things, choosing ways to do things and finding new ways

*It was your own idea to make the boat and to develop your storyline. At the end you started to extend your creative ideas and your story, putting the boat on its edge.*

**Child's comments:**

*You really enjoyed it when we looked through this Learning Story together and you started to tell me more too!*

**Parents' comments:**

*Eilish's parents love the story too and told me that she makes up her own stories all the time at home.*

**Possibilities and opportunities (what next?):**

*We will plan to extend your interest in using materials to create objects that you are then able to use for your storytelling. Perhaps you would be interested in using story props too to retell your stories? We will also plan more opportunities for you to use clay.*

## Activity

### A Learning Story

For the next observation you make on a child, try out the format used in the examples of Learning Stories in this chapter. Write in the first person and write it as if to the child. Begin your story with "I saw you …" and in the next section, What it means, start with "I think this means you …" If you are a student, share it with your mentor/supervisor before you share it with the child, and ask if you can have permission to share it with the child's parents. If you are a practitioner, make sure you share it with the room leader or manager before sharing it with the child or parents.

## William's parent consultation meeting

### William, 20 months

William has now been in the setting for two months, and the settling-in review took place after his first few weeks. Parent consultation meetings take place once every three months. These are arranged at a time to suit the parents, once the key person has made their most recent summary of the records. It takes place in a quiet space and is of course additional to the informal daily discussions.

### Parent/carer observations and views

What does your child enjoy doing at home?

William likes books, baby dolls, toy fruit with velcro which he can cut with a knife is a favourite, playing with trucks and watching the *Charlie and Lola* television programme.

*What do you think your child enjoys most about their nursery experience?*

William enjoys the freedom of making a mess, socialising, exploring the textures of the environment and painting. He loves the big spaces indoors and out and the big garden too. He loves exploring.

### Child's views

His favourites at present are trucks, diggers and lorries.

### Key person's observations and views

What do you feel are the child's favoured activities/experiences?

Imaginative play of many kinds. William loves the trains, baby dolls and loves playing in the home corner. He really enjoys it when we have real vegetables in the home corner. He enjoys hide-and-seek games, exploring the environment, especially the big garden. He is making lots of vocal sounds and interacting with other children older and younger than him. He loves the sensory books and the sensory room, puppets, cornflour, other messy play.

### Next steps

William is making a lot of vocal sounds and chats away, and some recognisable words are emerging, as shown in the Learning Stories we have collected. We will continue to support and encourage his speaking, by talking with him and giving him plenty of stories using story props and puppets. We will begin to involve him in cooking activities and tabletop games, where there is lots of repeated language. We will take him on more visits to the big garden.

## What the experts say
### Observing children to evaluate your own practice

### Reggio Emilia

In Chapter 15, part of a poem by Loris Malaguzzi, the founder of the famous Reggio Emilia Preschools in Italy, was quoted. The practice in these preschools is generally recognised because of its exceptional quality, and is an influence on early years practitioners around the world. The practitioners respect and value the children as highly competent learners and see themselves as partners with the children, nurturing and guiding them.

Their observations of the children help the staff to reflect on their own practice and what to do next to extend their learning. They use their observations to document not only the children's thinking, learning and development, but also their own. "Documentation becomes a tool for teacher research, reflection, collaboration and decision making" (Malaguzzi, 1993).

## Vivian Gussin Paley

Someone who has influenced me most in working with young children, because of her deep understanding of children and how they think and learn, is Vivian Gussin Paley. Her work was discussed in Chapter 6 (see page 90). Each day she reflected on what she recorded and used this to evaluate what she and her assistants should do to improve their practice. In *The Boy Who Would be a Helicopter: The Uses of Storytelling in the Classroom* (Paley, 1991), she tells us: "Every day after the children leave, my assistants and I clean up quickly so we have time to compare revelations ... We speak of surprises, seldom of certainties. We want to talk about what we don't understand and what has not worked out according to expectations." Her assistants find this the most useful approach. We can also take up this idea. Observing the children helps us to observe our own practice because it helps us understand the children better and therefore helps us to develop our practice to better suit the children.

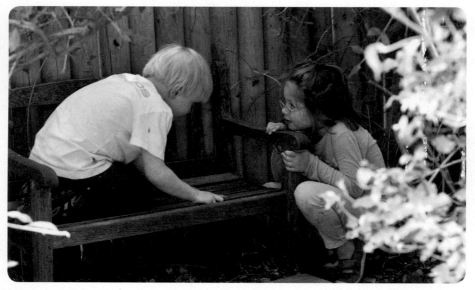

**Figure 16.5** Playing at being cats: observation leads to revelations about children's learning through play

# Effective practice:
## What do we need to do?

### Formative ongoing assessment

- Be observant and listen well. This will help ensure your interaction with the child is more likely to support their learning.
- Use a mix of methods for observing children, as set out in this chapter, depending on what your role is at the time.

- Note what is significant to the children's learning – what is new and different. Not everything needs to be written down. Remember the importance of interacting with the children.
- Carry out one planned and focused observation every three months (or each term, ensuring you analyse it to make the assessment). This could be more frequent, if necessary, for younger children or those with special needs.
- Always plan on the basis of what you find out.
- Share your observations with parents and children. Follow the processes set out in this chapter.

## Summative assessment

- Summarise your observations and assessments regularly to ensure that children are making progress in their learning and development. Keep track of progress. This can be done by using Development Matters as this provides a useful 'map', of what learning might look like.
- Carry out the 2-year-old progress check in a way that suits your parents and your setting, making sure you fulfil the statutory requirements. It is useful to include the Characteristics of effective learning too, as in Example 2 of the 'Know How Guide' (2012).

### Case study: Making it happen

At St Anne's Nursery School and Children's Centre there is a long-term plan and a termly plan, which sets out what the nursery wants children to be learning over the term. From this, a weekly plan is drawn up, but at this stage it is just an outline for the week, allowing for plenty of flexibility to amend and adapt according to what has happened. It is added to day by day.

A key part of planning is the daily planning meeting, which takes place for 15 minutes at the end of every day. At this meeting the day is evaluated, the children's learning is discussed and plans are adapted and fine-tuned for the next day to ensure the needs and interests of the children are met. This, too, is when the adult role is planned: who will be doing what, where and when the following day.

Each week, three children in each class group become the focus children for the week and all staff note down any new significant achievements – anything new and different they see the children do or say. The children are looked at in this way in rotation, but children with particular needs will be looked at more frequently. The observations are then collated into the children's records (at St Anne's they call these profiles) and next steps are drawn up. These children are discussed at the daily planning meetings to ensure the planning provides the necessary learning opportunities, building on their interests and introducing new ideas and interests, to support the children's next steps. The observations are shared with the children and the parents, and parents are encouraged to share them with their children too.

## Chapter summary

This chapter will have helped you:
➤ understand more about effective processes for ongoing formative assessment and the observation, assessment and planning cycle
➤ how and why to summarise children's learning in their learning and development
➤ understand how observation and assessment are at the heart of effective planning in the EYFS and how they will support you in creating the best for the children.

## Further reading and references

Carr, M. (2001) *Assessment in Early Childhood Settings: Learning Stories*, Paul Chapman Publishing, London

Drummond, T. (2010): http://tomdrummond.com/learning-stories/

Hutchin, V. (2007) *Supporting every child's learning in the EYFS*, Hodder Education, London

Malaguzzi, L. (1993) 'No way. The hundred is there' in *The Hundred Languages of Children: The Reggio Emilia Approach to Early Childhood Education*, Edwards, C., Gandini, L. and Forman, G. (eds.), Ablex Publishing Corporation, Norwood, NJ

Paley, V.G. (1991) *The Boy Who Would be a Helicopter: The Uses of Storytelling in the Classroom*, Harvard University Press, Harvard

### Useful websites

Early Education (where Development Matters can be found or bought at cost): www.early-education.org.uk

Learning Stories: http://earlylearningstories.info/
www.unisanet.unisa.edu.au/staff/SueHill/Learningstories.pdf

Reggio Emilia, Research into Practice, University of British Columbia, Vancouver: http://earlychildhood.educ.ubc.ca/community/research-practice-reggio-emilia

The Statutory Framework for the EYFS and 'A Know How Guide. The EYFS progress check at age two' can be found at: www.foundationyears.org.uk/early-years-foundation-stage-2012/

# Conclusion: Using the EYFS to reflect on and develop your practice

This book has taken you on a journey through all aspects of learning and development in the Early Years Foundation Stage 2012. This will have helped you to understand the EYFS, and to reflect on and evaluate how well you and your setting support the learning and development of children. We have looked at the implications for practice from crucial research and theory about learning, development and best practice. We have also looked at observations of many different children at different ages, at different points in their own learning journeys.

## Inclusive practice

We began in the first chapters with the EYFS principles and themes, and those important 'commitments'. These provide an important guide to effective practice and are a very useful tool for evaluating practice. How to ensure your practice is truly inclusive is one of the main themes woven through every chapter in this book. As a Statutory Requirement, inclusion and inclusive practice are key parts of the EYFS. Inclusion is highlighted in the principles and commitments of the **Unique Child** and **Learning and Development**, as well as underpinned by the principles and commitments of **Positive Relationships** and **Enabling Environments**. The **Development Matters** non-statutory guidance begins with a statement about the United Nations Convention on the Rights of the Child, emphasising at the outset the right of every child to have their needs fully met.

To demonstrate the uniqueness of every child and how best to support them, this book has provided over 50 observations of young children from a few weeks old to age 5. These show the differences and similarities in children's particular interests, in the ways they learn, and in their stages of development. They also show how careful analysis of observations has helped the practitioners who work with the children and their parents to support the children in their learning and development.

These observations are included in this book to support you in reflecting on and evaluating your own practice. Is every child equally well supported – whatever their starting points and stage of development? Do your records of children's learning and development show that all children are progressing well? What more can be done?

## Positive Relationships: how are children being supported in their learning and development?

A fundamental theme in this book has been that it is the quality of interaction between adults and children which is at the heart of effective practice. This entails knowing when to interact and when to stand back. It begins with observing and listening before joining in. And the key person is of course 'key' in the support for the child. Are all children in your setting well supported through positive relationships?

Partnership with parents is another important theme woven throughout this book. Positive relationships between practitioners and parents are vital in supporting children's learning and development: how successful are the relationships with parents in your setting?

## Enabling Environments: do the experiences you provide respond to children's individual needs?

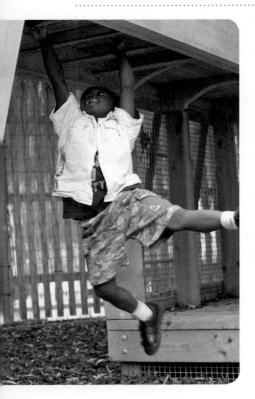

This book has provided many activities to help you to review and evaluate your environment, to ensure it is meeting children's needs. It also includes many examples of how practitioners have ensured their settings are enabling. Does the environment you create enable all children to learn and develop? Children learn *so much through* their own self-initiated activities and play, and the environment for play and exploration is an important teacher.

Let us end by looking at two more children whose own drive to explore and learn has been supported by their parents and practitioners, enabling them to develop and progress.

### Ernest

Ernest is now 5 years old and in a reception class in a maintained infants' school. This is the end of his second term in reception. As he has been blind since birth, he not only has a special support assistant with him at all times in school, but the staff in school and his parents at home receive regular support and advice from the specialist visual impairment teacher who visits him regularly. The focus of support from his assistant since he started school has been to help him gain confidence, help him to find his way around an unfamiliar environment, build his gross and fine motor skills, and to join in with all the learning experiences other children are accessing.

As a result of the support he is getting from his parents and the school, he is making rapid progress and is well aware of the progress he is making. With support, he has been involved in the wide range of first-hand experiences that all the other children are involved in – and more besides, to meet his needs. He is already making big strides in literacy, and is able to help other children to find the initial letter sounds of words. He is also beginning to read some Braille letters and is learning to track along the Braille with his fingers, and use the Brailler. He has made special friends with some other children, and one observation shows him joining in dancing with another child. On his first walk down to the end of the garden, he says "Look I CAN do it!" and he was even more pleased when Sarah, his assistant, told him: "I'm so proud of you Ernest!" He has recently begun to use a cane, and observations show him describing what he identifies: the rubber mat at the door, stairs, the carpet, a chair and the table.

## Sofia

Sofia began in a nursery setting at 3 years old. Over her first few weeks, she enjoyed playing in the home corner, at the mark-making table, and in the book corner, especially if an adult was there reading stories. Although her key person was really pleased about her development in mark-making and interest in reading, she was also aware that Sofia seemed anxious about going outside and only chose to go when her key person was outside and had encouraged her to come too.

Sofia had few opportunities to play outside at home, as her mother was also caring for her own disabled mother. Sofia's mother was keen for her to feel more confident outside. During the next few months, with support and encouragement from her key person and other practitioners, Sofia's confidence outside grew. Soon, she was joining others in the sandpit, as well as in the role play area. Her key person encouraged her to try the climbing equipment too, and to join in making an obstacle course.

One day her key person set up a mini beast hunt, following the interests of other children. She invited Sofia to join in. These hunts continued throughout the summer months. Sofia very quickly became one of the mini beast 'experts' in the group, telling others the names of the creatures they found, observing them, drawing them, taking photographs and contributing to the books the nursery made about mini beasts.

Along with all the other children whose observations appear in this book, with the help and support from the practitioners in their settings, both Ernest and Sofia's confidence as capable, competent and resilient learners had grown, ensuring their development in all areas of learning.

# Appendix: Early Learning Goals

## The Prime Areas of Learning and Development

### Communication and language

**Listening and attention:** Children listen attentively in a range of situations. They listen to stories, accurately anticipate key events, and respond to what they hear with relevant comments, questions or actions. They give their attention to what others say and respond appropriately, while engaged in another activity.

**Understanding:** Children follow instructions involving several ideas or actions. They answer 'how' and 'why' questions about their experiences and in response to stories or events.

**Speaking:** Children express themselves effectively, showing an awareness of listeners' needs. They use past, present and future forms accurately when talking about events that have happened or are to happen in the future. They develop their own narratives and explanations by connecting ideas or events.

### Physical Development

**Moving and handling:** Children show good control and co-ordination in large and small movements. They move confidently in a range of ways, safely negotiating space. They handle equipment and tools effectively, including pencils for writing.

**Health and self-care:** Children know the importance of physical exercise and a healthy diet for good health, and talk about ways to keep healthy and safe. They manage their own basic hygiene and personal needs successfully, including dressing and going to the toilet independently.

### Personal, social and emotional development

**Self-confidence and self-awareness:** Children are confident to try new activities, and say why they like some activities more than others. They are confident to speak in a familiar group, will talk about their ideas, and will choose the resources they need for their chosen activities. They say when they do or don't need help.

**Managing feelings and behaviour:** Children talk about how they and others show feelings, talk about their own and others' behaviour, and its consequences, and know that some behaviour is unacceptable. They work as part of a group or class, and understand and follow the rules. They adjust their behaviour to different situations, and take changes of routine in their stride.

**Making relationships:** Children play co-operatively, taking turns with others. They take account of one another's ideas about how to organise their activity. They show sensitivity to others' needs and feelings, and form positive relationships with adults and other children.

## The Specific Areas of Learning and Development

### Literacy

**Reading**: Children read and understand simple sentences. They use phonic knowledge to decode regular words and read them aloud accurately. They also read some common irregular words. They demonstrate understanding when talking with others about what they have read.

**Writing:** Children use their phonic knowledge to write words in ways which match their spoken sounds. They also write some irregular common words. They write simple sentences which can be read by themselves and others. Some words are spelt correctly and others are phonetically plausible.

### Mathematics

**Numbers:** Children count reliably with numbers from 1 to 20, place them in order and say which number is one more or one less than a given number. Using quantities and objects, they add and subtract two single-digit numbers and count on or back to find the answer. They solve problems, including doubling, halving and sharing.

**Shape, space and measures:** Children use everyday language to talk about size, weight, capacity, position, distance, time and money to compare quantities and objects and to solve problems. They recognise, create and describe patterns. They explore characteristics of everyday objects and shapes, and use mathematical language to describe them.

### Understanding the world

**People and communities:** Children talk about past and present events in their own lives and in the lives of family members. They know that other children don't always enjoy the same things, and are sensitive to this. They know about similarities and differences between themselves and others, and among families, communities and traditions.

**The world:** Children know about similarities and differences in relation to places, objects, materials and living things. They talk about the features of their own immediate environment and how environments might vary from one another. They make observations of animals and plants and explain why some things occur, and talk about changes.

**Technology:** Children recognise that a range of technology is used in places such as homes and schools. They select and use technology for particular purposes.

## Expressive arts and design

**Exploring and using media and materials:** Children sing songs, make music and dance, and experiment with ways of changing them. They safely use and explore a variety of materials, tools and techniques, experimenting with colour, design, texture, form and function.

**Being imaginative:** Children use what they have learned about media and materials in original ways, thinking about uses and purposes. They represent their own ideas, thoughts and feelings through design and technology, art, music, dance, role play and stories.

# Index